Cultural Competency for Health Administration and Public Health

Patti R. Rose, MPH, EdD

University of Miami
Visiting Assistant Professor
Coral Gables, Florida

JONES AND BARTLETT PUBLISHERS
Sudbury, Massachusetts
BOSTON   TORONTO   LONDON   SINGAPORE

2011

World Headquarters

Jones and Bartlett Publishers
40 Tall Pine Drive
Sudbury, MA 01776
978-443-5000
info@jbpub.com
www.jbpub.com

Jones and Bartlett Publishers
Canada
6339 Ormindale Way
Mississauga, Ontario L5V 1J2
Canada

Jones and Bartlett Publishers
International
Barb House, Barb Mews
London W6 7PA
United Kingdom

Jones and Bartlett's books and products are available through most bookstores and online booksellers. To contact Jones and Bartlett Publishers directly, call 800-832-0034, fax 978-443-8000, or visit our website, www.jbpub.com.

Substantial discounts on bulk quantities of Jones and Bartlett's publications are available to corporations, professional associations, and other qualified organizations. For details and specific discount information, contact the special sales department at Jones and Bartlett via the above contact information or send an email to specialsales@jbpub.com.

This publication is designed to provide accurate and authoritative information in regard to the Subject Matter covered. It is sold with the understanding that the publisher is not engaged in rendering legal, accounting, or other professional service. If legal advice or other expert assistance is required, the service of a competent professional person should be sought.

Production Credits

Publisher: Michael Brown
Editorial Assistant: Catie Heverling
Editorial Assistant: Teresa Reilly
Production Manager: Tracey Chapman
Senior Marketing Manager: Sophie Fleck
Manufacturing and Inventory Control
   Supervisor: Amy Bacus
Composition: DSCS/Absolute Service, Inc.

Cover Design: Kristin E. Parker
Cover Image: © Julian Fletcher/Dreamstime.com
Printing and Binding: Malloy, Inc.
Cover Printing: Malloy, Inc.

Library of Congress Cataloging-in-Publication Data
Rose, Patti Renee.
   Cultural competency for health administration and public health / Patti Rose.
      p. ; cm.
   Includes bibliographical references and index.
   ISBN-13: 978-0-7637-6164-6 (pbk.)
   ISBN-10: 0-7637-6164-8 (pbk.)
   1. Transcultural medical care. 2. Health services administration. 3. Cultural competence.
I. Title.
   [DNLM: 1. Cultural Competency. 2. Health Services Administration. 3. Public Health Practice.
W 21 R797c 2011]
   RA418.5.T73R67 2011
   362.1—dc22
                                  2009044575

6048
Printed in the United States of America
14 13 12 11 10   10 9 8 7 6 5 4 3 2 1

Dedication

I lovingly dedicate this work to my husband, Jeffrey Rose, and our children, Courtney and Brandon Rose, whose presence has given my life deep meaning and purpose and filled it with love and pride.

Table of Contents

Preface

In my roles in the field of health as a professor, consultant, writer, health service administrator, and researcher, I became keenly aware of the need for cultural competence in health service administration and public health. My awareness actually peaked while teaching at a university in south Florida where a majority of the students (master's of public health and medical) and faculty were from the mainstream population in the United States. In exploring where many of the students planned to practice after completing their degrees, namely communities comprised of minorities (south Florida and most major cities in the United States are very diverse), discussions led to the fact that they had limited or no insight into the cultures of those they planned to serve and their curriculum did not address this deficit.

Consequently, as a faculty member, I was asked to develop a series of lectures on various aspects of culture to supplement the curriculum of the medical and public health students. This led to my exploration of the Culturally and Linguistically Appropriate Services (CLAS) standards in health care, which were released by the Office of Minority Health (OMH) of the Department of Health and Human Services (DHHS) in December of 2000 (OMH DHHS, 2000). Additionally, in an effort to further enhance my cultural knowledge and to gain more insight before, during, and after the cultural competence lectures, I traveled to many countries in Latin America (the Dominican Republic, Cuba, Puerto Rico [a US territory], Mexico), Central America (Costa Rica, Nicaragua, Guatemala, and Belize), the Caribbean (Jamaica, the Virgin Islands, the British Virgin Islands, and Aruba), Africa (Kenya, Senegal, South Africa, and the Cape Verde Isles), Fiji, Japan, Sri Lanka, and Europe (Spain, the Netherlands, Corsica, Portugal, France, and Italy). My travels and extensive study led to an enhanced understanding of various cultures and cultural nuances.

A particularly interesting turning point for me as I proceeded with this travel and study, was the reading of a book titled *The Spirit Catches You and You Fall Down* in which Fadiman (1997) states:

> There are no funds in the hospital budget specifically earmarked for interpreters, so the administration has detoured around that technicality by hiring Hmong lab assistants, nurse's aides, and transporters, who

are called upon to translate in the scarce interstices between analyzing blood, emptying bedpans, and rolling postoperative patients around on gurneys. . . . Obstetricians have had to obtain consent for cesarean sections or episiotomies using embarrassed teenaged sons, who have learned English in school, as translators. Ten-year-old girls have had to translate discussions of whether or not a dying family member should be resuscitated. (p. 25)

The Spirit Catches You and You Fall Down is a compelling story of the suffering of a Hmong child with epilepsy within the American healthcare system. The incidents of linguistic and cultural incompetence that took place, negatively impacting the provision of health care for the child, are very disheartening. The idea that one's health care could be compromised because of a lack of understanding of one's culture and the inability to communicate with patients/clients/customers by healthcare and public health professionals seems implausible but is often a reality.

As described by Reynolds (2004):

The care that Lin receives leads to misdiagnosis and eventual decline in health care status as a result of communication barriers and lack of understanding from both the Lee family and her providers. Fadiman's account allows the reader to begin to understand dimensions of the Hmong cultural identity and the challenges that the U.S. health care system faces in adequately addressing the health needs of a defined population. (p. 241)

Furthermore, the lack of cultural competence in health care and public health is not only a problem in terms of language barriers (linguistic competence) for people who arrive in the United States from other nations to seek care but is also a problem for Americans who are born and raised in the United States and who only speak English. Take my mother, for example. Many years ago (she is now deceased), she became gravely ill. One of her primary illnesses was diabetes. Her doctor and nutritionist strongly encouraged her to change her diet and were quite firm with her when she failed to comply. Her doctor and nutritionist requested that a family member accompany her for her next visit, and I was selected by my mother to escort her. During this visit, I explained to her doctor and nutritionist, upon hearing their concerns, that although she lived in New York City and had done so for most of her adult life, she had been reared in Georgia and, consequently, her diet was primarily soul food, which she preferred. I further explained that she enjoyed cooking and prepared meals based on recipes that had been passed on in her family for many generations. The doctor and nutritionist asked me why she never told them this when they insisted that she change her diet. When I asked my mother why she did not tell them, she simply responded by saying, "They did not ask me." I proceeded to explain to the doctor and nutritionist, who were both white Americans, that soul food has a historical basis and was composed, in terms of its origin, of the remnants left by the slave masters after they ate the best parts of meat and the finest of all foods for their meals. The slaves took the scraps that were provided by their masters and turned them into tasty, highly seasoned dishes (often with a high salt content). Since my mother was an African American and a descendant of slaves, as most African Americans are, these dishes became a staple of her diet. The problem is that soul food is generally high in salt, fat, and sugar and includes frying as a mainstay of the preparation process. My suggestion to her doctor and nutritionist (as well as to my mother) was that she modify her diet rather than change it completely because the foods she ate and prepared were a significant cultural norm for her. Asking her to do otherwise was creating a serious cultural barrier and was leading to noncompliance, stress, and lack of communication that was exacerbating her overall health rather than helping her. This explanation helped in her care at the time because it promoted understanding and appreciation by her nutritionist and doctor regarding her food choices.

There is a great deal of miscommunication between patients/clients/customers and people in health care at various levels (staff and providers) and public health. The United States made a solid, concrete step toward improving the efficacy of health care and public health when, as mentioned earlier, the OMH released the CLAS standards. These 14 standards are guidelines, recommendations, and mandates aimed at ensuring that patients/clients/customers who seek care are treated with dignity, respect, and understanding in terms of their cultural and linguistic needs.

In reviewing these standards and other relevant topics and relating the information specifically to health services administration and public health, I have attempted to make this book, which provides an overview of cultural competence, a comfortable read with straightforward, comprehensible, and specific details. I believe that there are specific and important responsibilities that health service administrators and public health practitioners must meet in the provision of service and information. Therefore, it is imperative that healthcare executives and public health practitioners develop plans and initiatives to ensure that this occurs.

REFERENCES

Fadiman, A. (1997). *The spirit catches you and you fall down*. New York: Farrar, Straus and Giroux.

Office of Minority Health, Department of Health and Human Services. (2000). National standards on Culturally and Linguistically Appropriate Services (CLAS) in health care. *Federal Register, 65*, 247. Retrieved March 6, 2008, from http://www.gpo.gov/fdsys/pkg/FR-2000-12-22/pdf/00-32639.pdf.

Reynolds, D. (2004). Improving care and interactions with racially and ethnically diverse populations in healthcare organizations. *Journal of Healthcare Management, 49*(4), 241.

Acknowledgments

I came to realize during the writing of this textbook that the saying "no man is an island," or in this case "no woman is an island," is a valid statement. To that end, I would like to acknowledge my gratitude to a number of individuals who made this work possible. First, I begin with Vincent Omachanu, who provided excellent expertise for the establishment of reliability and validity of the cultural competence assessment surveys that comprise the first three appendices of this book. His expertise during our work on the survey project was offered with kind and expert assurance, and I thank him for that. I would also like to thank my colleague, Dr. Anthony Munroe, the former CEO of Economic Opportunity Family Health Center, Inc., in Miami, Florida, now aptly entitled the Jessie Trice Center for Community Health. During my tenure at the center as a Cultural Competence Consultant and subsequently as Vice President of Behavioral Health Services, I was able to implement a cultural competence action plan with his approval and with an excellent administrative team. This was an excellent opportunity to see the positive impact that cultural competence has when implemented correctly by health services administration and the implications for public health organizations.

Additionally, I would like to express my thanks to Dr. Edmund Abaka, Director of the Africana Studies Program at the University of Miami. Through his efforts to expand the program and create a rich learning experience for students, he offered the opportunity for the development of new courses that I was ready and willing to handle in the capacity of adjunct and then visiting assistant professor, a role that I currently hold in his program along with a joint appointment in American Studies. The new courses that are relevant to this text are *Black Women in Medicine and Healing*, *Race and Health Care in America*, and *Culture, Race and Diversity*. These courses enable discourse around the topic of cultural competence with an opportunity to provide insight to interested and enthusiastic students. I also thank my former research assistants, Stephanie Fenton and Paulo Pires, for their efforts. I am grateful for their assistance and acquisition of information relevant to this text.

I am grateful to Dr. Patrick Williams, who served as a sounding board, encourager, and ardent taskmaster. His understanding of the process of preparing this text was profound because he was completing his dissertation at the University of Miami at the time of my writing, so there was substantial opportunity for critical analysis based on similar intellectual tasks. Furthermore, I express my great appreciation to my excellent Barry University health services administration students, namely the Miami Children's Hospital cohort, for their excellence in my seminar course entitled *Cultural Competence in Health Services Administration*, a new course that I was asked to develop and teach. It enabled intense discourse on the subject of cultural competence and the opportunity to delve deeply with health service administrators who have the capacity to implement cultural competence initiatives in their work environment. Hence, I want to thank Dr. Alan Whiteman, Chair of the Department of Health Services Administration, for affording the opportunity for me to teach such outstanding master's level students.

Finally, but with the utmost gratitude and appreciation, I acknowledge my family, especially my husband, Jeffrey Rose, whose patience with my intensity regarding this project was profound and another example of the calm, fortitude, and strength that he provides for all endeavors in my life. I appreciated most his willingness to listen, his reading and proofreading of drafts, and his patience; this was yet another venture in our wonderfully adventurous life. I also acknowledge and thank my daughter, Courtney Rose, who recently graduated (June 2009) with a Master's Degree in Education from Harvard University. She not only understands the importance of cultural competence, but it was also an important aspect of her research while pursuing her degree because she feels it is extremely relevant to the field of education, and I agree. Hence, her thoughtfulness and intelligent conversation when I needed to explore ideas for inclusion in the textbook were quite helpful and insightful. I also thank my son, Brandon Rose, who recently graduated from Yale University (May 2009) with a Bachelor's Degree in History and who began law school at the University of Florida in 2009. His words of encouragement were extremely helpful, even as he struggled through the intensity of writing his senior essay while I was writing this book. Again I found a kindred spirit endeavoring in a similar task of writing. I wholeheartedly thank my family because, as with all that I do, it is for my wonderful husband and our amazing children, who are now young adults; I pursued this task knowing how much they believe in me and I in them.

Lastly, and with the highest regard, I thank God, without whom nothing I achieve would be possible.

About the Author

Dr. Patti Rose acquired her Master's Degree (MPH) in Health Services Administration from the Yale University School of Public Health followed by her Doctorate (EdD) in Health Education from Columbia University, Teachers College. She is currently a Visiting Assistant Professor for the University of Miami (UM) Africana and American Studies Programs for which she has developed new courses entitled *Black Women in Medicine and Healing, Race and Healthcare in America, African Women in the Diaspora,* and *Contemporary Issues in America.* Formerly, she served as CEO of Rose Consulting, Inc., followed by CEO of Plainfield Health Center in Plainfield, NJ. Prior to that she served as Vice President of Behavioral Health Services at Economic Opportunity Family Health Center (EOFHC), Inc., one of the largest community health centers in the nation, located in Miami, FL, and as a consultant for EOFHC. She has also held the title of Lecturer for the Yale University School of Public Health, Adjunct Professor for the UM Education Department and Executive MBA Program and for the Barry University Health Services Administration Program, Associate Professor at Nova Southeastern University in Fort Lauderdale, FL, and Assistant Professor at Florida International University in Miami, FL (graduate level public health programs). Her professional affiliations have included the American College of Health Care Executives, the American Public Health Association, the Black Executive Forum, and the National Association of Health Services Executives. She was inducted into the Public Health Service Honor Roll at the Yale University School of Public Health for her long-term commitment to public health service and was appointed by the US Department of Commerce, National Institute of Standards and Technology to serve in the capacity of Examiner on the 2004 Board of Examiners of the Malcolm Baldrige National Quality Award. Dr. Rose has been married for 24 years and is the mother of two young adults.

Chapter 1

Introduction

Overall, the purpose of this text is to explore in depth, at an introductory level, a good, solid rationale for healthcare administrators, public health practitioners, and students in the professions of health services administration and public health to consider the development of robust cultural competence plans as a necessity for enhancing the provision of quality care and as a business imperative. In this text, it is recommended that healthcare organizations and public health entities develop a cultural competence plan, akin to a business plan, recognizing the different needs and perspectives of the internal and external communities served. The result will be coordinated processes and policies that facilitate improved outcomes, improved patient satisfaction, mitigation of malpractice, and increased market share leading to an increase in the fiscal bottom line of healthcare and public health organizations.

It appears that the United States is going to embark on some type of healthcare reform. What it will ultimately consist of is unclear at this time. The current administration, under the leadership of President Barack Obama, is wrestling with this monumental task while the nation is watching the process unfold. The reform process has led to a national debate that is warranted. One significant consideration that needs to be included as part of the various aspects of healthcare reform is cultural competence. Although cultural competence is one of the initiatives of the US Department of Health and Human Services (DHHS) Office of Minority Health (OMH), as will be discussed in this text, it should become an intricate aspect of health service administration and public health as part of the fabric of every organization. Just as electronic medical records (EMRs) are needed to ensure that medical errors are reduced, cultural competence initiatives are needed to reduce malpractice claims and enhance customer service, as well as address other ongoing concerns. This book serves as a mere starting point for students, health service administrations, and public health practitioners to consider cultural competence as an imperative, but hopefully, cultural competence will become a significant component of the healthcare reform agenda.

American society appears ready for change and cultural competence. Recently, Congress formally apologized for the enslavement of African American people in the United States. Furthermore, for the first time in American history, the nation has an African American serving as President of the United States and an Hispanic woman serving as a Supreme Court Justice. Additional firsts for this nation include an African American Attorney General and an Asian American Secretary of Energy. Diversification is taking place at high levels in the United States, but this alone is not sufficient. There are still serious issues pertaining to race, communication, and cultural understanding in the United States. A specific example occurred when a prominent African American professor, Dr. Henry Louis Gates, Jr., who is the director of the W.E.B. Dubois Institute for African and African American Research/Studies at Harvard University, was arrested in his home by a White police officer. Per the media, a report of a potential burglary of Dr. Gates's home was phoned in to the police department by a neighbor of Dr. Gates. There was no burglary, as Dr. Gates was the person attempting to get into his home with his driver after he returned home from a long journey from China where he was conducting research. The ensuing communication between Dr. Gates and the police officer, who arrived at Dr. Gates's home to investigate the alleged burglary, went awry after Dr. Gates allegedly showed two forms of identification and established that it was in fact his home, leading to the arrest of Dr. Gates. Subsequently, Dr. Gates accused the officer of racial profiling, and the officer accused him of disorderly conduct. The result has been a nationwide discussion of racial issues in the United States that has included a comment by the President of the United States from his vantage point as an African American person.

Furthermore, the recent incident which occurred in January 2010, when the book by *Atlantic Reporters* Mark Halperin and John Heilemann, entitled *Game Change* was released, involving comments made by the Senate Majority Leader, Harry Reid during the 2008 Presidential campaign, led to a firestorm of debate and discussion. As indicated in the *Game Change*, Harry Reid stated that President Obama would win over John McCain, because he is "light skinned" and has no "Negro dialect." This racially insensitive comment led to requests for Senator Reid to step down from his Senate leadership position, a statement from President Obama and intense debates within all forms of media. These particular occurrences are clear indications that, specific discussion needs to continue to occur regarding the topics of race, culture, ethnicity, sensitivity, and diversity, among others.

The question that has surfaced since the election of the first African American President of the United States and African American First Lady of the United States is whether a postracial society has been accomplished. Former President Carter stated that he believes the current upheavals associated with healthcare reform in terms of rallies and town meetings, at which harsh signs have appeared depicting President Obama as a Nazi (Hitler) and other unsavory characters, are a result of racism toward President Obama because he is African American. During an interview on *NBC Nightly News* on September 15, 2009, with the television network anchor, Brian Williams, former President Carter stated the following:

> I think an overwhelming portion of the intensely demonstrated animosity toward President Barack Obama is based on the fact that he is a black man, that he's African American. I live in the South, and I've seen the South come a long way, and I've seen the rest of the country that share the South's attitude toward minority groups at that time, particularly African Americans. That racism inclination still exists. And I think it's bubbled up to the surface because of the belief among many white people, not just in the South but around the country, that African-Americans are not qualified to lead this great country. It's an abominable circumstance, and grieves me and concerns me very deeply.

Additionally, assassination threats toward President Obama are up 400%, according to several news establishments, including Cable News Network (CNN), and there has been an actual call for his death from a White minister. Although all are not in agreement with former President Carter's assessment, if he is accurate, then the United States has not achieved the goal of becoming a postracial society, and the need for ongoing dialogue about issues pertaining to race and culture becomes imperative.

This need for discussion and dialogue is relevant to health care and public health, because it is necessary to ensure that skill sets are in place, from a cultural vantage point, to deal with the rapid demographic changes and to close the long-standing health disparity between minority groups and White people. Specifically, if full-fledged cultural competence efforts are realized in the context of healthcare reform efforts, patients/clients/customers, many of whom are minorities, will be better served, which will lead to improved quality of care. Cultural competence is imperative and in our nation's best interest in terms of the provision of efficacious health care and public health.

The key questions pertaining to this text are as follows: What is cultural competence, and why is it relevant to health care, particularly in terms of health services administration and public health? Although the United States has never been a homogeneous population, the makeup of the population is changing as a result of immigration patterns and increasing birthrates among racially, ethnically, culturally, and linguistically diverse groups. The number of people who speak languages at home other than English has also increased dramatically. The foreign-born population in the United States has increased substantially, with the most rapid growth among Hispanics, which is now the largest minority group. African Americans/Blacks, formerly the largest minority group, are now a close second. Hispanics are an ethnic group, based on the language spoken (Spanish), but the primary language spoken is what distinguishes Hispanics from mainstream America. Therefore, the data associated with the increase in the number of Hispanics in the United States, and the number of Blacks and Whites (and other groups), are confounded because of the fact that Hispanics may be White or Black (or other) in terms of race. Consequently, perhaps their increasing numbers should be allocated in terms of race, not ethnicity, because this is how other groups are categorized in the United States. For example, Haitians speak Creole but are generally identified and categorized as Black in terms of race and not as a distinct group based on the language they speak. Granted, their numbers are much smaller, but it is not their language that is used to identify them in the United States, but their race, which is further delineated by their nationality (Haitian).

Nevertheless, the trend of an increasing number of minorities in the United States is expected to continue, which is leading to the use of the term *emerging majority*. The emerging majority includes all groups of minorities as established by the Office of Management and Budget (OMB) of the US government. OMB establishes the racial and ethnic categories in the United States, which, in terms of minorities, are African Americans/Blacks (race), Hispanics (ethnicity), Asian/Pacific Islanders (race), and Native Americans and Alaska Natives (race). Therefore, it is imperative that the provision of health care take place in a culturally competent manner in an effort to meet the needs of the emerging majority (ever increasing collective of minority groups) in the United States.

Additionally, there have been numerous approaches and attempts to define cultural competence. Linguistic competence has also been defined, which is equally important in ensuring optimal health care. Early in this text, a clear and cogent definition of this term will be provided, as offered by the OMH of DHHS, that takes both cultural and linguistic competence into consideration. OMH has also developed a significant initiative to address these concerns, and thus, an overview explaining why healthcare organizations must function in the context of respect and responsiveness to the cultural diversity of communities and patients/clients/customers served is also provided in this text. The effort to establish the necessity for cultural and linguistic competence and diversity was initiated in December of 2000 when the OMH released the Culturally and Linguistically Appropriate Services (CLAS) standards in health care. There are a total of 14 standards comprising mandates, guidelines, and recommendations. These standards are delineated and reviewed in this text. Furthermore, a clear distinction is made between the terms cultural competence and diversity. Often, the notion of ensuring cultural competence within healthcare administration and public health is considered to be the same as diversifying healthcare organizations, which is clearly inaccurate, although the need for diversity is explored and established as necessary to the same degree as cultural and linguistic competence. This concept of cultural and linguistic competence and diversity as three important and distinct necessities is clarified and thoroughly explained.

Furthermore, the role of healthcare administrators and public health officials is to plan and implement cultural competence within organizations in compliance with CLAS, state, federal, and accreditation requirements. Healthcare organizations increasingly rely on private accreditation entities, such as the Council on Education for Public Health (CEPH) and The Joint Commission, to set standards and monitor compliance within them. Cultural and linguistic competence is emerging as an important aspect of the accreditation process for healthcare organizations. Cultural competence is also relevant to healthcare organizations from a fiscal vantage point because it makes business sense. If healthcare patients/clients/customers are receiving care and services that are attentive to their cultural and linguistic needs and provided by a diverse staff that is reflective of those who are being served, they are more apt to use or return to a given facility and share their enthusiasm with others in their communities. In addition, malpractice claims will be reduced as result of enhanced cultural and linguistic communication.

There are a number of books that are currently available that address the topics of cultural competence, linguistic competence, cultural proficiency, diversity, and other related matters of concern. Some of these texts include descriptions and details about the various minority groups in the United States, their health concerns, and existing health disparities. What distinguishes this text from the others is the provision of details about minority groups that will enable service providers to appreciate, value, and understand specific insights about various cultures. For example, in Chapter 2, there is discussion regarding the most appropriate term to use in regard to ethnic and racial groups in the United States. Is it best to use the term Black or African American or both? Is it most appropriate to use the term Native American or Indian when communicating with indigenous American people? Although these questions do not have definitive answers because of their complexity and individual preferences, insight is provided as to the origins of the terms, giving helpful information that will prove useful in decision making as to whether one should use one term over the other when communicating with patients/clients/customers. This is an important detail because it is part of the culture of people of African descent and indigenous Americans, and failure to understand and use the appropriate terminology may prove to be problematic when serving them.

Furthermore, this book endeavors to explore the aforementioned designation of the Hispanic population as an ethnic rather than a racial group by the OMB, as mentioned previously. When one encounters an Hispanic person in a healthcare or public health setting, it is pertinent to determine their race and nationality because the nation that a person who speaks Spanish comes from will determine his or her culture, not the fact that he or she speaks Spanish. As an example, in viewing the literature regarding the new Supreme Court Justice, Judge Sotomayer, the preponderance of literature referred to her as the first Hispanic nominee. Although this is true, what is her race? Is she White, Black, Asian, or Native American? Given that she is also from Puerto Rico (a US territory), how does she differ culturally from other Hispanics who are not from Puerto Rico but perhaps from the Dominican Republic, Guatemala, or Honduras? The term Latina was often used in discussions about her in the media. What is the difference between the terms Hispanic and Latino(a)?

Such inquiry matters in health care and public health because differences in culture based on nationality/lineage impact health-seeking behavior, diet, communication, and other relevant factors that are necessary to understand to provide optimal service. Often, data pertaining to Hispanics are strictly reported under the category of Hispanic without any detail regarding race or nationality. This is problematic because categorization of health data for Hispanics should include Black Hispanics under the Black/African American racial category and White Hispanics under White, and so forth, without exception, because Hispanics may be from any of the four racial groups determined by OMB.

Again, for each racial category, insight should also be provided regarding nationality because of the distinct cultural differences among the nations where people have their lineage. For example, a person from Nicaragua does not have the same cultural background as a person from the Dominican

Republic, although they both may speak Spanish, and a Black person from Jamaica has a very different cultural background from a Black person from Trinidad or from the United States. If dietary habits are considered, as an example, from a cultural perspective, there is significant variation, and hence, data regarding the various groups' health problems associated with dietary habits would have to reflect such differences. Thus, it is incorrect and culturally inappropriate to report data collectively on the health status of Black people, Asian people, Hispanic people, and Native American people without these considerations of nationality and cultural differences. Therefore, the intention of this book is to ensure that the reader understands the nuances of culture and what is necessary to know in ensuring culturally competent service. Ultimately, cultural competence is not only the right thing to do from an appropriate and altruistic vantage point but a business imperative, particularly with the significant, rapid, and continuous changes in the diversity of those served.

CHAPTER ORGANIZATION

This book contains 11 chapters, including this Introduction. There are learning objectives, key terms, conclusions, chapter summaries, chapter problems, references, and suggested readings within each chapter, beginning with Chapter 2. All key terms appear with definitions throughout the text and in the glossary at the end of the book. Also, at the end of the book are cultural competent attitudinal assessment surveys (for health services administrators, staff, and providers); a list of pertinent Web sites, journal articles, and books (from the past and present); a sample cultural competence plan; and an index for the reader's convenience.

Chapter 2

Cultural Competence and Diversity: Is There a Difference?

LEARNING OBJECTIVES

After reading this chapter you should be able to:

- Define cultural competence and other key terms.
- Differentiate between cultural competence and diversity.
- Understand rapid demographic changes in the United States.
- Delineate key racial and ethnic groups in the United States including African Americans/Blacks, Asians/Pacific Islanders, Native Americans and Alaska Natives, Whites, and Hispanics.
- Recognize the significance of cultural competency and why it is imperative for healthcare organizations and public health.

KEY TERMS	
Culture	Ethnicity
Cultural competence	Linguistic competence
Cultural filtration	Nationality
Diversity	Race
Emerging majorities	

INTRODUCTION

There is a distinct difference between the concepts of cultural competence and diversity, although they are often used interchangeably. This chapter will explore those differences by reviewing the terms and discussing strategies to increase cultural competence and diversity as separate but interrelated entities. It is essential to explore current and projected demographics pertaining to the majority and minority groups in the United States. Through this exploration, a basis is established for the fact that cultural competence is an imperative for health service administrators and public health practitioners to ensure optimal services to all people as they interact with and seek services from those individuals who serve in these fields.

DEMOGRAPHIC CHANGES

There are currently significant demographic changes taking place in the United States that are having a direct impact on healthcare organizations and public health. Per the US Census Bureau, minority populations grew dramatically from 1980 to 2000 from 20% to 31%, respectively (Hobbs & Stoops, 2000). Traditionally, the United States has always been known for diversity based on an influx of individuals from all over the world. Table 2-1 provides recent detail regarding foreign-born residents.

Kosoko-Lasaki, Cook, and O'Brien (2009) provide statistics in regard to specific groups of undocumented immigrants:

> In the 1900's an estimated 350,000 undocumented immigrants entered the United Sates in 2004, 81% were from Latin America, 9% from China, 6% from Europe and Canada, and 4% from Africa and other countries. Children under 18 years of age (1.7 million) accounted for 17% of the undocumented population in 2004. (p. 255)

Additionally, Kosoko-Lasaki et al. explain the refugee population:

> according to the United Nations, a *refugee* is a person who, "owing to a well founded fear of being persecuted for reasons of race, religion, nationality, membership in a particular social group, or political opinions outside the country of his nationality, and is unable to or owing to such fear, is unwilling to avail himself of the protection of that country." More than 2 million refugees were admitted to the United States between 1975 and 2000. (p. 255)

Table 2-2 provides insight in terms of the number of refugees in the United States.

Often, the goal of immigrants was to seek greater opportunities beyond their homelands. This is true for practically all groups found in the United States that are not indigenous populations, with the exception of African

Table 2-1 Foreign-Born Residents, 2000

Statistic	Value
Total US population, 2000	281,421,906
Foreign-born population, 2000	31,107889
Percentage of residents who were foreign born, 2000	11
Percentage of foreign-born population who arrived 1900–2000	43
Percentage of foreign-born population in 2000 from top five countries of origin	
Mexico	30
China	5
Philippines	4
India	3
Vietnam	3
Percentage of foreign-born population in 2000 by region	
Latin America	52
Asia	26
Europe	16
Africa	3
North America	3
English proficiency	
Percentage of the total US population ages 5 or older with limited English proficiency	8
Percentage of foreign-born population ages 5 or older with limited English proficiency	51

Source: US Department of Homeland Security, US Citizenship and Immigrant Services, Office of Citizenship. (2004). *Helping immigrants become new Americans: Communities discuss the issues.* Retrieved November 8, 2009, from http://www.uscis.gov/files/article/focusgroup.pdf. Also see US Census Bureau at http://quickfacts.census.gov.

Americans, who were brought in captivity as slaves by Europeans as chattel to work the land.

Diversity in American society has made it necessary to understand the healthcare needs of various groups in an effort to provide optimal services and to understand health-seeking behaviors, attitudes, cultural nuances, and perceptions about health. This discussion begins with an exploration of cultural competence, its meaning, and why it is imperative as an undertaking for healthcare organizations and public health.

Table 2-2 Statistics on Refugees in the United States

Area	Period	Number
Africa	1980–2000	Total >85,000; >30,000 Ethiopian; 25,000 Somali; the remainder Sudanese, Liberian, Zairian, Rwandan, Ugandan, and Angolans
Southeast Asia	1975–2000	Total >1.4 million; ~900,000 Vietnamese; the remainder Laotian, Cambodian, and Burmese
Near East, South Asia	1980–2000	Total 112,500; ~47,000 Iranian; ~31,200 Iraqi; ~28000 Afghan
New Independent States and the Baltic	1989–2000	Total >378,000
Former Soviet Union	1989–2000	Total 546,516
Yugoslavia	1992–2000	Total ~107,000
Latin America	1975–2000	Total 79,634

Source: US Department of State, Bureau of Population. (2000). *Refugees and Migration, January 18, 2000*. Retrieved November 8, 2009, from http://www.state.gov/www/global/prm/admissions_resettle.html#fact; Refugee health: Immigrant health. Background on refugees. (2004). Retrieved November 8, 2009, from http://bearspace.baylor.edu/Charles_Kemp/www/refugees.htm.

CULTURAL COMPETENCE

In recent years, cultural competence has become a significant concept in health care and public health. In some settings, it generates controversy because of concerns regarding its necessity and cost-effectiveness. To many, it is a misunderstood concept that does not seem to have relevance to health services administration and public health. Thus, it is important to spend some time exploring the definition of cultural competence. The overriding definition of **cultural competence**, as there are many, is provided by the Office of Minority Health (OMH) of the US Department of Health and Human Services (DHHS), which states that, "Cultural and linguistic competence is a set of congruent behaviors, attitudes, and policies that come together in a system, agency, or among professionals that enables effective work in cross-cultural situations" (US DHHS, 2005).

LINGUISTIC COMPETENCE

Linguistic competence involves understanding the fact that many people in the United States do not speak English or have limited English proficiency and seek health care in environments where their predominant language is not spoken; hence, there is a need for linguistic competence in the provision of health care and public health to ensure effective communication. Unfortunately, many individuals who do not speak English do not receive optimal care because of language barriers. The definition of **linguistic competence** per the National Center for Cultural Competence at Georgetown University is as follows:

> The capacity of an organization and its personnel to communicate effectively, and convey information in a manner that is easily understood by diverse audiences including persons of limited English proficiency, those who have low literacy skills or are not literate, and individuals with disabilities. (Goode & Jones, 2004)

There are numerous languages other than English that are spoken in the United States, as indicated in Figure 2-1.

Often, healthcare organizations will use interpreters to assist with language barriers. As stated by Kosoko-Lasaki et al. (2009):

> Medical interpreting is a specialty in high demand as healthcare as healthcare systems strive to improve language access. Healthcare systems from megahospitals to neighborhood clinics, develop language access plans to comply with governmental regulations, attain facility certification, increase patient certification and improve public health. Plans include how and where to find language services including volunteers, bilingual staff, independent contractor interpreters and telephonic language bureaus. (p. 106)

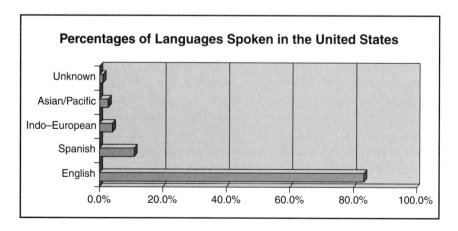

Figure 2-1 Languages other than English spoken in the United States.
Source: Data from United States Census, 2000.

The use of family members (particularly children) as interpreters can be a precarious situation because it is inappropriate (due to confidentiality or reversal of parent–child relationships, which is problematic in some cultures). It is also inappropriate to use nonclinical and bilingual staff because medical terminology may be misinterpreted by nonclinical staff and bilingual staff may confuse dialects/terms that are unique to a given culture. For example, regarding the latter, a word in Spanish spoken by a person from Costa Rica may not have the same meaning as the same word in Spanish spoken by a person from Puerto Rico. Therefore, to strive toward accuracy, it is only appropriate to use trained interpreters (either in person or by telephone). The use of untrained interpreters may also cause other problems beyond incorrect interpretation of words and concepts, including the wrong use of health-related terminology, the inclusion of personal perspectives in the interpretation process, and violation of confidentiality. The trained interpreter is aware of all of the possible errors mentioned and is better prepared to avoid them. The goal is to avoid **cultural filtration**, which is when cultural beliefs or ideas are either included or removed from the interpretation process by the interpreter. This can also occur in the process of translation of written materials (Reynolds, 2006).

DIVERSITY, RACE, AND ETHNICITY

It is important to distinguish the concept of cultural competency from that of diversity. For the purpose of this discourse, **diversity** refers to the makeup of the workforce of a given healthcare organization. This includes ethnic and racial backgrounds, age, physical and cognitive abilities, family status, sexual orientation, socioeconomic status, religious and spiritual values, and geographic location (Betancourt, Green, & Carillo, 2002). The United States is a very diverse nation consisting of a predominant or majority group (the White population) and minority groups, including African Americans/Blacks, Hispanics, Native Americans and Alaska Natives, and Asians/Pacific Islanders. The White group is considered the majority population based on their larger percentage of the total population in the United States, and the remaining groups are viewed as minorities because of their smaller percentages. It is important to note that Whites, African Americans/ Blacks, Native Americans and Alaskan Natives, and Asians/Pacific Islanders are racial groups, whereas Hispanics are an ethnic group. **Race** refers to "biological variation including phenotypical differences in stature, skin color, hair color, facial shape and other inherited characteristics that may or may not be mutually exclusive in each individual" (University of Wisconsin–Fox Valley, 2006). **Ethnicity** refers to "a group or individual's conception of cultural identity which includes a wide variety of learned behaviors that a human being uses in his or her natural and social environment to survive which may result in cultural demarcation between and within societies" (University of Wisconsin–Fox Valley, 2006).

Hispanics/Latinos

Hispanic is an ethnicity rather than a race based on the fact that one can be White Hispanic or Black Hispanic; White or Black serves as the racial identity, and Hispanic serves as the ethnic identity. Essentially, people who identify their origin as Hispanic or Latino may be of any race. Therefore, the percentage of Hispanics or Latinos should not be added to percentages for racial categories. Hispanics can be further classified by **nationality**, which is an identity that can be defined by a person's place of legal birth or by a person's associational citizenship status governed by where an individual resides and works, which may defy national boundaries and sovereignty (Borak, Fiellin, & Chemerynski, 2004). *Hispanics or Latinos* are those people who classify themselves in one of the specific Spanish, Hispanic, or Latino categories listed on the Census 2000 questionnaire, namely "Mexican, Mexican American, Chicano," "Puerto Rican," or "Cuban," as well as those who indicate that they are "other Spanish/Hispanic/Latino."

Persons who indicate that they are "other Spanish/Hispanic/Latino" include those whose origins are from Spain, the Spanish-speaking countries of Central or South America, or the Dominican Republic or people identifying themselves generally as Spanish, Spanish American, Hispanic, Hispano, Latino, and so on. Table 2-3 provides detail regarding the sociodemographics pertaining to this group. Again, people who identify their origin as Spanish, Hispanic, or Latino may be of any race, with commonality based on the language spoken, that is, Spanish. The various groups that comprise the Latin American population are listed in Table 2-4.

Although the terms Latino and Hispanic have been used interchangeably for decades, experts who have studied their meanings say the words trace the original bloodlines of Spanish speakers to different populations in opposite parts of the world. Hispanics derive from the mostly White Iberian Peninsula that includes Spain and Portugal. Latinos are descended from the brown indigenous Indians of the Americas south of the United States and in the Caribbean, who were conquered by Spain centuries ago. Furthermore, the term Hispanic was given prominence during the Nixon administration more than 30 years ago through the Office of Management and Budget (OMB) (Fears, 2003). The term appeared not only on census forms, but also on all other federal, state, and municipal applications for employment, general assistance, and school enrollment.

Table 2-3 Sociodemographic Characteristics of Hispanics

Characteristic	Value	
Hispanic or Latino (2006)	47.5 million	
In the 50 states	43.7 million	
Commonwealth of Puerto Rico	3.8 million	
Population not Hispanic or Latino	255.4 million	
Total US population (50 states) (2006)	299.1 million	
Hispanic subpopulations (2006)		
Mexican Americans	66.0%	
Puerto Ricans	9.4%	
Central Americans	7.8%	
South Americans	5.2%	
Cuban Americans	4.0%	
Other Hispanics	7.6%	
	Hispanic Whites	**Non-Hispanic Whites**
Age		
Median age, Hispanics (2007)	27.4 Years	40.5 Years
≥65 years (2005)	6%	15%
Education, completed high school or more (2004)	58.4%	90%
Income: families with annual earnings <$35,000	50.9%	26%

Sources: US Census Bureau. (2006). *2005 Puerto Rico survey* (B03002-3-est). Washington, DC: Author; US Census Bureau. (2004). *The Hispanic population in the United States: March 2004*. Retrieved November 8, 2009, from http://www.census.gov/population/www/socdemo/hispanic/ho04.html; US Census Bureau. (2004). *Current population reports: Educational attainment in the United States, detailed tables (PPL-169)*. Retrieved November 8, 2009, from http://www.census.gov/population/www/socdemo/education/cps2004.html; US Census Bureau. (2007). *Annual estimates of the population by sex, race, and Hispanic or Latino origin for the United States: July 1, 2006 (NC-EST 2006-04)*. Retrieved November 8, 2009, from http://www.census.gov/popest/states/asrh/SC-EST2006-04.html; US Census Bureau. (2005). *65+ in the United States: 2005*. Retrieved November 8, 2009, from http://www.census.gov/prod/2006pubs/p23-209.pdf; and US Census Bureau. (2004). *Current population survey, 2004 annual social and economic supplement*. Retrieved November 8, 2009, from http://www.census.gov/apsd/techdoc/cps/cpsmar04.pdf.

African Americans/Blacks

African Americans/Blacks are now the second largest minority group in the United States, after a long-held position as the largest minority group. Per the Office of Minority Health and Health Disparities (2009), "the African American population is represented throughout the country, with the greatest concentrations in the Southeast and mid-Atlantic regions, especially Louisiana, Mississippi, Alabama, Georgia, South Carolina and

Table 2-4 Percentage of Racial and Ethnic Groups in Latin America

Racial/ Ethnic Group	Mestizo (%)	Mulatto (%)	Mixed (%)	Amerindian (%)	White (%)	Black (%)	Other (%)
Mexico	60			30	9		1
Cuba		51			37	11	1[a]
Columbia	58	14			20	4	
El Salvador	90			1	9		
Brazil	53.7	38.5				6.2	1.6
Peru	37			45	15		3[b]
Guatemala	59.4[c]			40.6[d]			

[a] Chinese.

[b] Indigenous peoples (Mayans) including K'iche (9.1%), Mam (7.9%), Q'eqchi (6.3%), other Mayans (8.6%), and others (0.3%).

[c] Mestizo and European.

[d] Blacks, Japanese, Chinese, and others.

Source: Central Intelligence Agency. (2009). *The world factbook*. Retrieved September 17, 2009, from https://www.cia.gov/library/publications/the-world-factbook/docs/profileguide.html.

Maryland." Blacks have been referred to by many titles in the United States, including Colored, Negro, Black, Afro-American, African American, and other terms, not mentioned here, that are considered derogatory. These varying terms used to describe people of African descent in the United States were largely derived within political and historical contexts. Specifically, the term Colored was used as a result of the following:

> The 1924 law restricting immigration might be the pivotal one here. . . . The first ever comprehensive immigration restriction law—with a racial and national hierarchy that favored some immigrants over others. . . . This immigration law treated race as obvious and visible as it split the world up into "colored" and "non-colored" races, and into European and non-European. (Ruben and Melnick, 2006, p. 8)

The term Negro has a different origination. One speculative perspective follows:

> Let us look back into history, then, and strive to discover the origin of this term "Negro." If you look at the unabridged edition of the Oxford Dictionary, you will be shown that the origin of the word "Negro," as far as is known in the English language, is in 1555. Nevertheless, that is not the beginning of the term because the English were not the first transgressors in this respect. The English adopted the word from the Spanish. The Spanish may have gotten it from the Portuguese; it isn't yet quite clear. (Moore, 1992, p. 35)

The term Afro-American was used to describe Blacks of African descent, and there are many theories regarding its origin, some of which follow per Herbst (1997).

> Although sometimes said to date from the early 1850s, Flexner (1976) dates it to the 1830s and says it was used largely by Northerners or applied to free black people during the era of enslavement. Mencken (1962) cites a black leader, Dr. Kelley Miller, who in 1937 argued that *Afro-American* was coined in 1880 by T. Thomas Fortune, editor of *Age*. Miller also claimed that in the early twentieth century an English explorer of Africa, Sir Harry Johnston, shortened Afro-American to *Aframerican*, suggested perhaps, as Mencken (1962) notes, by the coinage *Amerindian*; but Aframerican was never very popular. In any case, *Afro-American* was revived by the 1960s. (p. 4)

By the late 1980s, the term Afro-American was largely superseded by African American. However, Afro-American is still used by the Library of Congress for cataloguing purposes and is also retained in names of organizations or programs, such as Yale University's Afro-American Cultural Center.

Additionally, many still use the term Black, which is historically inaccurate (Spivey, 2003). According to Spivey, "Ninety Percent of all African Americans have their ancestral roots in the kingdoms of West Africa" (p. 53). Consequently, the term African American is used to make a connection to this ancestral lineage, which is historically correct. In July of 2009, the President of the United States, Barack Obama, and his wife, Michelle Obama, and their two children visited Ghana, the first nation to gain independence in Africa. While there, President Obama and his family visited Elmira Castle, which was the largest slave-holding facility on the continent of Africa. Other such castles exist, including one that stands today near Senegal on Goree Island which this author had the opportunity to visit. These castles are remnants and tangible evidence of the transport of African slaves from West Africa to the New World, which we know today as the United States of America. Some may prefer Black as a more unifying term because they may identify themselves as persons from specific nations, such as Jamaican American, Trinidadian American, and so on. In these instances, African is not the lead term, although they are also of African descent. Others will solely use their nationality to describe themselves, indicating, for example, that they are Jamaican or Haitian and leaving out the term American even if they were born in the United States but are descendants of parents born in Jamaica, Trinidad, and so on.

Native Americans and Alaska Natives

The notion of nationality as a key element of understanding culture applies to all of the groups mentioned earlier. However, Native Americans (labeled as American Indians by the OMB), who have been identified as indigenous to the United States, have a nationality that is unequivocally American. Other terms have been used to identify them, including Indian, but some are considered derogatory. As Ruben and Melnick (2006) explain:

> Writing in 1941, an Indian immigrant to the United States named Krishnalal Shridharani wrote, with tongue in cheek, about Columbus's "discovery" of America: "We Hindus take a pardonable pride in the fact that had it not been for us 'undiscovered' Indians, America would not have been the same America from 1492 on. (p. 139)

This refers to the fact that Native Americans were given the title Indians because when Christopher Columbus arrived in the Americas during his exploratory voyages, he thought that he was in India and hence incorrectly named the Native people "Indians." Therefore, use of the term Native American is preferred and appropriate for many from this racial group. Furthermore, Native American groups should not be equated with other ethnic minorities. The fact is that Native American tribes—by treaty rights—own their own lands and have other rights that are unique to the descendants of the real natives of America. No other minority within the United States is in a similar legal position. Native peoples view themselves as separate nations within a nation. US laws and treaties, officially endorsed by US presidents and the Congress, confirm that status (Lanouette, 1990).

Furthermore, due to the unfortunate history of how Native Americans have been treated in the United States, as stated in Kosoko-Lasaki et al. (2009) in terms of "past segregationist practices, inferior housing and physical environments . . . disenfranchisement, extermination of tradition, language and land rights; broken treaties; sterilization of Native women . . . and other experiences of oppression" (p. 230), there are a number of consequences that include, but are not limited to, intergenerational anger and grief as mistrust of government. Additionally, "treatments provided in a culturally insensitive manner are ineffective. . . . Health care must recognize and comply with Natives' values, beliefs, and traditions in order to provide acceptable services (Kosoko-Lasaki et al., p. 230). Table 2-5 provides insight into some of the leading causes of death of Native American people.

Table 2-5 Leading Causes of Death Among Native Americans in 1980 and 2004

	2004		1980	
Ranking	Cause of Death	No. of Deaths	Cause of Death	No. of Deaths
	All causes	13,124	All causes	6,923
1	Diseases of the heart	2,598	Diseases of the heart	1,494
2	Malignant neoplasms	2,392	Unintentional injuries	1,290
3	Unintentional injuries	1,520	Malignant neoplasms	770
4	Diabetes Mellitus	746	Chronic liver disease and cirrhosis	410
5	Cerebrovascular disease	581	Cerebrovascular disease	322
7	Chronic lower respiratory diseases	486	Homicide	217
8	Suicide	404	Diabetes mellitus	210
9	Influenza and pneumonia	291	Certain conditions originating in the perinatal period	199
10	Nephritis, nephritic syndrome, and nephrosis	247	Suicide	181

Source: National Center for Health Statistics. (2006). *Health, United States, 2006. With chartbook on trends of the health of Americans.* Hyattsville, MD: Author.

Asian Americans and Pacific Islanders

Asian Americans are generally designated as people in the United States who are grouped not by language but because they arrived from Asia, namely from Vietnam, Indonesia, Japan, Korea, China, and other nations. Culturally, there are significant differences among these groups. One half of all immigrants in the United States since 1965 have come from Asia. Asian Americans have distinct notoriety in America as the "model minority" given their tendency to assimilate into the mainstream, from the vantage point of education, strict work ethic, and rapid grasp of the English language (Duncan & Goddard, 2005). They are one of the fastest-growing racial categories in the United States (Reynolds, 2006). Asian Americans are extremely diverse, coming from approximately 50 countries and speaking 100 different languages. According to Reeves and Bennet (2003):

> Ninety-five percent of all Asians and Pacific Islanders lived in metro-politan areas, a much greater proportion than of non-Hispanic Whites (78 percent). Of the two populations, Asians and Pacific Islanders were

twice as likely to live in central cities located in metropolitan areas (41 percent compared with 21 percent). However, among those living in metropolitan areas but not in central cities, Asians and Pacific Islanders were only 3 percentage points below non-Hispanic Whites (54 percent and 57 percent, respectively). (p. 2)

THE IMPORTANCE OF CULTURAL COMPETENCY FOR HEALTHCARE ORGANIZATIONS AND PUBLIC HEALTH

With the earlier provision of examples of the significance of terminology used to describe various minority groups, at least two of the groups, Blacks and Hispanics, combined with the other minority groups, are leading to **emerging majorities**. This term is used to describe an inevitable change taking place in American society based on the prediction that by the year 2050, in certain geographic areas in the United States, the majority populations will be Hispanics and Blacks and other minorities (combined), and Whites will be the minority group. Therefore, understanding key aspects of Hispanics, Blacks, and other racial and ethnic groups is imperative in terms of the provision of health care and public health services. In particular, the main racial and ethnic groups, as described earlier and as determined by the OMB, are designated by category for federal statistics and administrative reporting (OMB, 1997). The categories determined by the OMB are delineated in Table 2-6. These categories are considered essential (although under intense scrutiny and criticism because some people feel that they do not reflect accurately the racial diversity of the US population) in terms of the provision of health care in the United States with specific attention focused on nationality and other aspects of individuals and their culture.

Culture

Depending on one's culture, there are nuances that may be significant to health-seeking behaviors, attitudes, diet, whom individuals prefer to receive care from, whether or not individuals will return for care, and so on. **Culture** is an integrated pattern of learned beliefs and behaviors that can be shared among groups. It includes thoughts, styles of communicating, ways of interacting, views on roles and relationships, values, practices, and customs (Robins, Fantone, Hermann, Alexander, & Zweifler, 1998; Donini-Lenhoff & Hendrick, 2000). Culture also includes a number of additional influences and factors, such as socioeconomic status, physical and mental ability, sexual orientation, and occupation (Betancourt et al., 2002).

Table 2-6 Office of Management and Budget, Racial and Ethnic Categories/Standards

Race	Description
American Indian or Alaskan Native	A person having origins in any of the original peoples of North America, and who maintains cultural identification through tribal affiliations or community recognition.
Asian/Pacific Islander	A person having origins in any of the original peoples of the Far East, Southeast Asia, the Indian subcontinent, or the Pacific Islands. This area includes, for example, China, India, Japan, Korea, the Philippine Islands, and Samoa.
African American/Black	A person having origins in any of the Black racial groups of Africa.
White	A person having origins in any of the original peoples of Europe, North Africa, or the Middle East.

Ethnicity	Description
Hispanic	A person of Mexican, Puerto Rican, Cuban, Central or South American, or other Spanish culture or origin, regardless of race.

Source: Office of Management and Budget. (1995). *Standards for the classification of federal data on race and ethnicity.* Washington, DC: Author.

It is essential that healthcare and public health organizations learn to meet the needs of individuals served; otherwise, optimal, efficacious care may not be provided. There are consistent reports indicating that there are racial and ethnic disparities in health. The Institute of Medicine (IOM) investigated such disparities in 2003 and provided concrete recommendations aimed at reducing them in a report entitled *Unequal Treatment: Confronting Racial and Ethnic Disparities in Health Care* (Smedley, Stith, & Nelson, 2003). Some of the recommendations included increasing awareness of such disparities, integrating cross-cultural education into the training of healthcare professionals, use of evidence-based guidelines to promote consistency and equity of care, and continued research to assess disparities further and provide appropriate interventions.

The IOM introduced a second report in 2004 entitled *In the Nation's Compelling Interest: Ensuring Diversity in the Health Care Workforce*, which focused on institutional and policy level strategies aimed at increasing diversity within the healthcare workforce (IOM, 2004). Although the focus of this report was diversification of the fields of medicine, nursing, and psychology, this is also necessary in the fields of health services administration and public health. Ensuring a diverse and culturally competent healthcare environment necessitates a top-down approach beginning with the board of directors, administrators, and public health officials. Failure to recognize the need for diversity at these levels may preclude an understanding of the inherent needs of specific racial and ethnic groups. Insight from leaders who are representatives of ethnic and racial minority groups and who understand the need to diversify the workforce at every level in health services administration and public health may prove to be extremely helpful in delivering efficacious health care for the individuals and populations served.

STUDENTS

To ensure a racially and ethnically diverse workforce in health services administration and public health, the process has to begin with educational institutions and students. The first step is to ensure that students who are representative of racial and ethnic minority groups are admitted to programs that will train them to work in these fields. Additionally, healthcare administration and public health curriculums must include information about racial and ethnic health disparities, cultural competence, diversity, and the rapid change in demographics in the United States. Additionally, assessment must take place to identify any biases and stereotypes that students may hold that may preclude their ability to develop and implement comprehensive and effective cultural competence plans in their respective work environments. Health services administration and public health schools, departments, and programs must include research that focuses on health disparities, cultural competence, and diversity issues, and they must understand that failing to do so will negatively impact the quality of care provided to patients and, ultimately, the fiscal bottom line of healthcare organizations and public health entities.

FISCAL ACCOUNTABILITY AND CULTURAL COMPETENCY

Without cultural competence, the fiscal bottom line of healthcare and public health organizations may be impacted because cultural groups may decide not to use facilities that do not service them appropriately and hence the facilities lose market share. This is particularly true as diversity continues to expand in the United States and varying racial and ethnic groups grow larger in their respective communities and beyond. Although there is a great deal of altruism involved in cultural competence and diversity within healthcare organizations, there is also a bottom-line aspect to moving in this direction. Healthcare administrators and public health officials are interested in optimal financial and strategic performance. Therefore, the need for cultural competence and diversity in healthcare organizations should be reflected in their directive strategies, which include the mission, vision, and values statements; policies; and strategic plans of organizations. The benefits for health service administrators and their organizations, and public health entities where appropriate, will include profitability based on maintaining and growing current and future market share, enhancing the reputation of healthcare and public health organizations with ethnic and racial minorities, developing a sustainable competitive advantage over organizations that are not proceeding with cultural competence and diversity efforts, improved customer service, motivation of staff as they experience better relationships with the individuals they serve, and ultimately enhanced productivity. Conceivably, these efforts would lead to earnings growth, acceptable return on investments (because there is an expense factor associated with cultural competence and diversity initiatives), and cost reduction over time. This aspect of the significance of cultural competence and diversity and the need for a paradigm shift will be discussed in greater detail in Chapter 3.

ACCREDITATION AND CULTURALLY AND LINGUISTICALLY APPROPRIATE SERVICES IN HEALTHCARE STANDARDS

Healthcare and public health accrediting organizations now require their respective fields to meet certain cultural competence accreditation requirements. These organizations include the Council on Education for Public Health (CEPH) and The Joint Commission. Furthermore, the Culturally and Linguistically Appropriate Services (CLAS) standards in health care, released in December 2000 by the OMH of the DHHS, were developed as clear guidance on how to provide culturally and linguistically appropriate services in healthcare settings. The accreditation requirements and the CLAS will be discussed at length in Chapters 9 and 10.

CONCLUSIONS

There is a need for a paradigm shift to accomplish the comprehensive process of incorporating cultural competence as a key component of health services administration and public health. This requires an investment of time, people, money, and information. There is also a need to diversify employees at every level in both fields based on race, nationality, ethnicity, and other key factors to ensure that these entities reflect the communities served in terms of their workforce at every level of the hierarchical structure of organizations. Linguistic competency is also imperative to ensure that no matter the language spoken by individuals, they will be served optimally within healthcare organizations and within the context of public health efforts. Healthcare organizations must ensure readiness in the area of cultural competence in terms of accreditation requirements for organizations such as CEPH, The Joint Commission, and others and adherence to CLAS. As stated by Betancourt et al. (2002), "In the end the ultimate goal is a healthcare system and workforce that can deliver the highest quality of care to every patient, regardless of race, ethnicity, cultural background, or English proficiency" (p. 2).

CHAPTER SUMMARY

The key reasons for cultural competence in health services administration and public health are to respond to current and projected demographic changes in the United States; to eliminate long-standing disparities in the health status of people of diverse racial, ethnic, and cultural backgrounds; and to improve the quality of services and health outcomes. These efforts will lead to greater customer satisfaction and appreciation of services and contribute to the improvement of the fiscal bottom line of healthcare organizations. Diversification of the workforce in health services administration and public health is also imperative with the understanding that cultural competence and diversity are distinctly different terms that should not be used interchangeably. Diversity and cultural competence are needed as separate but interrelated requirements.

CHAPTER PROBLEMS

1. Cultural competence and diversity are two distinct but interrelated terms. Explain the difference between the two terms and why both are relevant to health services administration and public health.

2. A patient, who speaks Spanish only, arrives at a healthcare facility for care with her 10-year-old son. A staff person, who speaks English only, arrives to greet the patient and realizes that the patient does not speak English and immediately asks the patient's bilingual (English and Spanish speaking) son to serve as interpreter. Explain whether or not the staff person took the correct approach in trying to communicate with the patient.

3. The president and chief executive officer (CEO) of a healthcare firm arrives at a meeting to provide information to the executive leadership about a new cultural competence initiative that will take place at the facility. He advises that every measure should be taken to keep costs down related to the effort because it is an altruistic venture for the organization but will not lead to any financial benefit. What type of tone about cultural competence is the president and CEO setting by disconnecting it from any level of financial benefit to the organization?

4. Public health workers are assigned to conduct research in a metropolitan community to determine potential reasons for obesity, diabetes, and other issues. The researchers are advised by their supervisor in a preparation meeting that although the community members comprise solely people who are Haitian or African American, there is no need to present the research findings on the two groups distinctively because all of the community members are all Black and hence their cultural and social characteristics, including diets and exercise habits, will be the same. Explain the problem(s), if any, with this directive.

5. A children's hospital in the United States has a contract to serve families from a small Arab-speaking nation who will fly in their children for specialty care when needed. The marketing director of the hospital advises his staff to develop a brochure for the incoming patients in English. One of the staff members objects, suggesting that the patients will not understand the brochure because they do not speak English. The marketing director responds by stating that, "If a patient wants to receive care here and read our informational materials, they better learn English and fast." Is there a problem with this director's perspective regarding the patients to be served, and does he need cultural competence or linguistic competence training? If so, describe possible approaches.

References

Betancourt, J. R., Green, A. R., & Carrillo, E. J. (2002). *Cultural competence in health care: Emerging frameworks and practical approaches.* New York: The Commonwealth Fund.

Borak, J., Fiellin, M., & Chemerynski, S. (2004). Who is Hispanic? Implications for epidemiologic research in the United States. *Epidemiology, 15*(2), 240–244.

Donini-Lenhoff, F. G., & Hendrick, H. L. (2000). Increasing awareness and implementation of cultural competence principles in health professions education. *Journal of Allied Health, 29*(4), 241–245.

Duncan, R., & Goddard, J. (2005). *Contemporary America* (2nd ed.). New York: Palgrave, Macmillan.

Fears, D. (2003, August 25). Latinos or Hispanics? A debate about identity. *The Washington Post*, p. A01. Retrieved March 26, 2008, from http://webhost.bridgew.edu/lasociedadlatina/articles/latinos%20or%20hispanics.pdf.

Goode, T., & Jones, W. (2004). *Definition of linguistic competence, National Center for Cultural Competence*. Washington, DC: National Center for Cultural Competence, Georgetown University Center for Child and Human Development. Retrieved February 24, 2008, from http://www11.georgetown.edu/research/gucchd/nccc/foundations/frameworks.html.

Herbst, P. (1997). *The color of words: An encyclopedic dictionary of ethnic bias in the United States*. Boston: Intercultural Press.

Hobbs, H., & Stoops, N. (2000). *Demographic trends in the 20th century. U.S. census bureau 2000 special reports, series CENS R-4*. Washington, DC: US Government Printing Office.

Institute of Medicine. (2004). *In the nation's compelling interest: Ensuring diversity in the health care workforce*. Washington, DC: The National Academies Press.

Kosoko-Lasaki, S., Cook, C., & O'Brien, R. (2009). *Cultural proficiency in addressing health disparities*. Sudbury, MA: Jones and Bartlett Publishers.

Lanouette, J. (1990). Native American stereotypes (teacher's corner). *Anthropology Notes, 12*(3), 1. Retrieved April 23, 2008, from http://anthropology.si.edu/outreach/Indbibl/sterotyp.html.

Moore, R. B. (1992). *The name "negro": It's origin and evil use*. Baltimore: Black Classic Press.

Office of Management and Budget. (1997). Revisions to the standards for the classification of federal data on race and ethnicity. *Federal Register* Notice, October 30. Retrieved February 22, 2008, from http://www.whitehouse.gov/omb/rewrite/fedreg/ombdir15.html.

Office of Minority Health and Health Disparities. (2009). *Black or African American populations*. Retrieved July 19, 2009, from http://www.cdc.gov/omhd/Populations/BAA/BAA.htm.

Reeves, T., & Bennett, C. (2003). *The Asian and Pacific Islander population in the United States*. Washington, DC: US Census Bureau.

Reynolds, D. (2006). Improving care and interactions with racially and ethnically diverse populations in health care organizations. *Journal of Healthcare Management, 49*(4), 243.

Robins, L. S., Fantone, J., Hermann, J., Alexander, G., & Zweifler, A. (1998). Improving cultural awareness and sensitivity training in medical school. *Academic Medicine, 73*(10 Suppl), S31–S34.

Ruben, R., & Melnick, J. (2006). *Immigration and American popular culture*. New York: New York University Press.

Smedley, B. D., Stith, A. Y., & Nelson, A. R. (Eds.). (2003). *Unequal treatment: Confronting racial and ethnic disparities in health care*. Washington, DC: The National Academies Press.

Spivey, D. (2003). *Fire from the soul of the African-American struggle.* Durham, NC: Carolina Academic Press, 53.

US Department of Health and Human Services. (2005). *What is cultural competency?* Retrieved February 20, 2008, from http://www.omhrc.gov/templates/browse .aspx?lvl=2&lvlID=11.

University of Wisconsin–Fox Valley. (2006). *An anthropological perspective of ethnicity and race.* Retrieved July 19, 2009, from http://www.uwfox.uwc.edu/academics/ depts/perspective.html.

SUGGESTED READINGS

Baxter, C. (2001). *Managing diversity and inequality in healthcare.* Oxford, UK: Bialliere Tindall.

Byrd, M., & Clayton, L. (2000). *An American health dilemma: A medical history of African Americans and the problems of race: Beginnings to 1900.* New York: Routledge.

Jones, D. (2006). The persistence of American Indian health disparities. *American Journal of Public Health, 96*(12), 2122–2134.

Naylor, L. (Ed.). (1997). *Cultural diversity in the United States.* Westport, CT: Bergin and Garvey.

Purnell, L., & Paulanka, B. (1998). *Transcultural healthcare: A culturally competent approach.* Philadelphia: F.A. Davis.

Richard, A. (Ed.). (2007). *Eliminating healthcare disparities in America.* New York: Humana Press.

Chapter 3

Health Service Administration and Public Health and the Paradigm Shift

LEARNING OBJECTIVES

After reading this chapter, you should be able to:

- Understand the need for a paradigm shift.
- Discuss cultural competence as a market-based issue.
- Understand how the implementation of cultural competence leads to the expansion of minority markets and may enhance the bottom line of organizations.
- Explain the need for a diverse workforce and health services administration.
- Understand aspects of necessary training in cultural competence for health services administrators and public health students.

KEY TERMS

Bottom line	Paradigm shift
Informed consent	Return on investment
Mainstream	Visual affirmation
Malpractice	

INTRODUCTION

To a large extent, although not exclusively, cultural competence is a market-based issue. Hence, to explore this in depth, the discussion of a need for a paradigm shift for healthcare organizations is necessary with an emphasis on approaches to expand minority markets and enhancement of the bottom line of organizations. A diverse workforce that has experienced appropriate cultural competence assessment and training can ensure an optimal environment of service and lead to positive outcomes. Students trained to work in the field of health services administration or public health must learn the importance of cultural competence in their respective fields and why it is necessary to run an effective organization from the vantage point of strategic planning, marketing, and enhanced customer service.

THE NEED FOR A PARADIGM SHIFT

A **paradigm shift** is "a revolutionary change from one way of thinking to another, which does not just happen but is driven by agents of change" (Waldren, 2004). This is necessary in American society in terms of moving health services administration and public health toward embracing the notion of cultural competence. Although the United States has never been a largely homogeneous society, the continued and rapid change in demographics is moving the society toward vast changes in its population. Therefore, understanding various communities in order to serve them efficaciously, in terms of health care, public health, and beyond, is imperative. In addition, such a paradigm shift is necessary in the healthcare field to expand minority markets and to improve the **bottom line** performance of organizations through enhancement of customer service and perhaps increasing the market share of those individuals from various cultures who appreciate and recognize the benefits of services designed to meet their cultural needs. The bottom line refers to the net income of an organization.

For a paradigm shift to take place, there has to be long-term and sustained commitment from the top down, beginning with the board of directors, the chief executive officer (CEO) and other administrators, providers, and staff. Actions must include the identification of barriers to culturally competent goals such as unwillingness on behalf of the organization to embrace such endeavors, concerns about costs associated with the process, and other issues that may arise in trying to move forward with change. Top-level commitment is an indication of seriousness and has a trickle-down effect for employees at all levels of organizations. Infrastructure change is also necessary, including the physical surroundings of healthcare organizations, such as artwork and images that reflect the patients/clients/customers served, which is referred to as **visual affirmation**. There must also be policies that reflect cultural competence, as a serious indication of the importance of the matter, as well as changes to other organizational directional strategies, including the mission, vision, and value statements, the strategic and marketing plans, and so on. Allocation of resources has to be determined to support cultural competence initiatives and the identification of benchmarks and rewarding of successes. Additionally, educational requirements in academic institutions that offer degrees in the areas of health services administration and public health must be initiated to ensure the opportunity to hire staff with adequate cultural competence levels/skills as well as diversification of the health service administration and public health workforce. In short, the process of achieving a paradigm shift is comprehensive and requires serious change.

EXPANSION OF MINORITY MARKETS

The first step in ensuring the expansion of minority markets is to begin with efforts to make sure that members of minority communities are aware that services are in place to meet their specific needs. This begins with marketing. As an example, advertisements and communication directed toward minority communities must be visually affirming and developed in terms of their language. Specifically, if advertisements are developed to target members of the African American community, images in the marketing material should include African American people. Advertisements for Hispanic communities should be multilingual (in both Spanish and English) to ensure language proficiency. There will likely be costs associated with the translation of such materials, but the initial investment is worthwhile to ensure optimal communication. This approach applies to all minority groups. Brochures and materials must be visually diverse, as a starting point, to attract customers by clearly enabling them to see themselves reflected in any outward communication. This process should not seem unusual to organizations that are approaching cultural competence seriously. Such apparent approaches to cultural competence, language proficiency, and diversity details (in terms of images) will serve to enhance the reputation of healthcare organizations with their patients/clients/customers because they will see themselves reflected in the environment where they receive or plan to receive health services.

Furthermore, healthcare organizations that embrace cultural competence, linguistic competence, and diversity will have a sustainable competitive advantage over organizations that maintain a monolithic approach to providing services. Healthcare organizations will not be successful if they continue to conduct business as if the demographics are not changing and under the belief that society only responds to mainstream images and approaches.

INVESTING IN CULTURAL COMPETENCE

Clearly, changes toward cultural competence require an expenditure of money or investment on efforts to revise key aspects of the organization, such as diversification, training, moving patient/client/customer environments toward culturally visual affirmation, demographic data analysis, and so on. However, the **return on investment** (ROI), which is the monetary benefit derived from having spent money on developing or revising a system, will be worth the effort. It will be hard to quantify the benefits of such endeavors because the results will often be long term and intangible. Nevertheless, through customer service surveys, demographic data to determine market share, increases and decreases in malpractice claims based on culturally biased events, and other factors, the evidence to support moving in the direction of cultural competence will surface.

In an effort conducted by IBM in 1995, the CEO, Lou Gerstner, took a radical approach that led to the turnaround of the company. He initiated efforts that considered workforce diversity as an area of strategic focus (Thomas, 2004). What was striking about this initiative is that Gerstner did not enact it for the sake of diversification only; he approached the process as a market-based issue in an effort to improve the organization's bottom line, and the outcome was, and continues to be, a great success. His efforts were not limited to diversification efforts only, but included cultural competence strategies and a clear understanding that the two terms, diversity and cultural competence, are not synonymous. The goal of the IBM effort was to minimize differences, which is often the opposite of what is seen in American society. Differences are often considered deviation from the **mainstream**, which is "a term that is often used to describe the 'general market,' usually refers to a broad population that is primarily white and middle class" (Smedley, Stith, & Nelson, 2003, p. 524). This type of thinking is extremely problematic in the healthcare arena because healthcare services and public health efforts often take place in communities that are very different from the mainstream. Organizations will benefit from targeted efforts at diversifying health care and public health, beginning from the top down and implementing cultural competence initiatives. A business case must be established for such action by taking a look at the intended communities to be served from a demographic perspective and targeting them accordingly with progressive positive approaches that have their optimal care and health needs in mind.

THE BUSINESS ASPECT OF HEALTH CARE

Although the purposes of health service and public health organizations are to serve those in need of preventive and curative services and to serve the community at large (focusing on entire populations rather than individuals), this does not preclude the notion that these organizations include a business aspect, which is the financial component of the provision of services. It costs money to provide health care and to conduct public health efforts. Services must be paid for, whether it is through health insurance, out-of-pocket payments, government or philanthropic sources, or other sources. Therefore, developing efforts that are reflective of those who are in need of the services makes good business sense. Consequently, healthcare administrators and public health officials must align their strategic business goals for their organizations with their diversity and cultural competence goals.

Thus, it is important for healthcare organizations to gain greater insight into their major markets at every level. Specifically, if a healthcare organization is located in a community that was largely mainstream in the past and that gradually or suddenly experienced an influx of a particular minority group or groups, it behooves the organization to establish a rapport with the changing community(s) on every level. This requires, first and foremost, learning about the culture of the communities and diversifying staff to reflect the community in an effort to ensure that customers feel compatible with those who will serve them. Additionally, it is important to communicate with individuals in their language to prevent a language barrier and to provide cultural competence training for all staff at every level. Training should include universal language techniques, rather than the requirement of learning additional languages, because learning additional languages would be an unreasonable requirement. Some universal language techniques are simple and include actions such as smiling upon initiating communication, which is a universal form of positive communication. Understanding matters regarding hand gesturing, eye contact, and touching, which vary between cultures, is an important aspect of universal communication. Training will also ensure that staff, taking culture into consideration, will be able to discern particular health needs and concerns and any barriers that may exist in terms of the provision of services. Once barriers are discerned, from a cultural vantage point, the organization will be better prepared to address them. By doing so, the organization gets closer to the community and vice versa, leading to a reciprocal relationship in which the community wants to maintain a long-standing relationship with the healthcare organization, primarily because the organization cares and is meeting the needs of the community. Given that the community will pay for services, in one form or another, and public health entities will benefit from serving the community, from a strict business vantage point and if providing optimal services to the community, the outcome is a win–win situation and perhaps a profitable venture, as indicated in Figure 3-1.

According to the National Center for Cultural Competence, there are a number of reasons to incorporate cultural competence into organizational policy, including greater market share, increased profits, and decreased malpractice issues (Cohen & Goode, 1999). One of the reasons highlighted is "gaining a competitive edge in the market place," which indicates the value of embracing cultural competence in order to position healthcare

Cultural Competence and Profitability

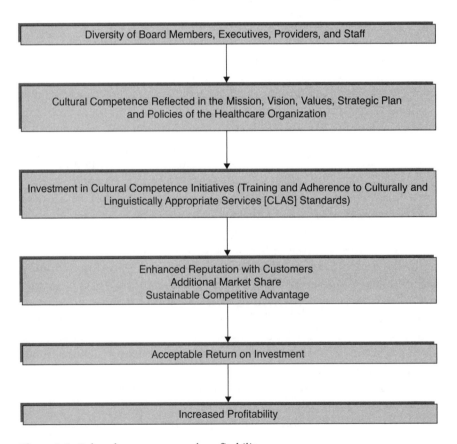

Figure 3-1 Cultural competence and profitability.

organizations to better handle the continued surge of diversity in the marketplace (Cohen & Goode, 1999). Health service administrators and public health officials must ensure that staff, at all levels, acquire cultural knowledge and skill sets that enable them to work with diverse populations. This is essential in the strategic planning process to seize opportunities for future growth as immigrants, minorities, and others continue to gain access to healthcare coverage and services. It is important to prepare for an ever-growing diverse population and to be able to communicate effectively to ensure an emphasis on two key components of the bottom line—increased market share and increased profits (Suro, 2000). This does not preclude the altruistic aspect of such an endeavor, which is to ensure optimal service because it is the right thing to do, but simultaneously recognizes that individuals from different cultures comprise a growing demand for health services and public health initiatives.

For example, a significant number of nonelderly Latinos in the United States are without health coverage (although many do have some kind of private insurance or Medicaid), and the number is growing. However, Asians and Pacific Islanders generally have coverage approaching that of Whites. Additionally, as immigrants continue to work their way into jobs with health benefits, the size of the market will increase exponentially (Suro, 2000). As an illustration of how the process may be handled, the following Robert Wood Johnson Foundation (RWJF) grant for a project entitled "Opening Doors" should be considered. The RWJF provided a grant in the amount of $4 million, which supported 23 projects in rural and urban areas in 11 states and demonstrated the following results:

- Reduction of unnecessary emergency room visits in a rural immigrant community
- Increased patient enrollment in an urban hospital-based health maintenance organization (HMO) where interpreters and outreach workers were available for immigrants
- HMO compliance with state standards for access to reproductive health care and cultural competence in managed care

These results were accomplished by using community outreach workers, providing interpreter services, changing policies and practices that created barriers to care, developing cross-cultural curricula for medical students, providing community-based training opportunities for residents, and offering cultural competence training for agency staff and board members. These accomplishments reflect a cost-effective endeavor (RWJF & Henry J. Kaiser Family Foundation, 1997).

DECREASING MALPRACTICE CLAIMS

Another reason for the provision of cultural competence that makes good business sense for a healthcare organization is to "decrease the likelihood of malpractice claims" (Cohen & Goode, 1999). **Malpractice** is improper or negligent treatment of a patient, as by a physician, resulting in injury, damage, or loss. Lack of awareness about differences and failure to provide interpretation and translation services may result in one or more of these occurrences and lead to liability in a number of ways. Healthcare organizations may also be liable due to failure to obtain **informed consent**, which is consent by a patient to a surgical or medical procedure or participation in a clinical study after achieving an understanding of the relevant medical facts and the risks involved. Failure to translate such a document for a non–English-speaking patient can lead to significant problems.

Additionally, failure to understand beliefs and practices may translate into breaches of professional standards of care or the presumption of negligence. Healthcare organizations must address linguistic competence, as a component of cultural competence, to ensure accurate and effective communication in languages other than English (Cohen & Goode, 1999). The ability to communicate effectively has been shown to reduce the likelihood of malpractice claims. A study in the *Journal of the American Medical Association* indicates that patients of physicians who were frequently sued had the most complaints about communication. The study identifies specific and teachable communication behaviors associated with fewer malpractice claims. Physicians can use these findings to decrease malpractice risks, and health service administrators can use them to ensure that their malpractice insurers provide this information to guide risk prevention (Levinson, Roter, Mullooly, Dull, & Frankel, 1997). This is particularly important because malpractice claims can be costly and may severely impact the bottom line of healthcare organizations and public health entities.

ENHANCED CUSTOMER SERVICE AND QUALITY OF CARE

There is no doubt that cultural competence is evolving from a marginal to a mainstream healthcare policy issue and as a potential strategy to improve quality and address disparities (Reynolds, 2004). Hence, health service administrators and public health practitioners must understand that cultural competence strategies and training, at all levels of organizations, will ensure an understanding of culture and respect for differences, allowing for more culturally effective planning and intervention decisions. Knowledge of specific cultures permits those involved in health services administration and public health to understand how to develop programs, treatment protocols, and interventions that are based on culturally based beliefs and can impact outcomes in a positive direction, leading to improved quality of care and better customer service. "Quality of care is reliant on an organization's ability to communicate effectively and understand the cultural factors that affect health behavior" (Reynolds, 2004, p. 246).

CONCLUSIONS

Embracing of cultural competence by health service administrators and the field of public health requires a paradigm shift. As the demographics of American society continue to change drastically, efforts toward serving diverse populations must be enhanced. There are a number of reasons for these efforts, but a significant factor is that market share will be expanded through greater outreach to minority markets, which may lead to an enhanced fiscal bottom line. Cultural competence should be included as part of the strategic plan and business aspect of healthcare organizations with hopes of a sustained competitive advantage over organizations that do not recognize the need for such efforts.

CHAPTER SUMMARY

The key goals at the core of cultural competence efforts, within the context of considering cultural competence as a component of the business aspect of health service organizations and public health entities, are visual affirmation; diversification of board members, executives, providers, and staff; avoidance of malpractice claims through effective communication; and enhanced customer service. All of these efforts will make a difference in the provision of services with an eye toward cultural competence.

Ensuring that patients/clients/customers and communities see themselves within the context of the environments where they are served and through the people who serve them will indicate to them that their needs have been considered and that services have been designed for them. This, in turn, will lead to the perception and hopefully the reality of enhanced customer service, new patients/clients/customers, and a desire for patients/clients/customers to return and spread the word about the services they receive. As a result, healthcare organizations can expect an enhanced bottom line due to increased volume.

CHAPTER PROBLEMS

1. A healthcare organization has an excellent waiting room area for its patients/clients/customers in need of emergency care and would like to redesign it to reflect the clientele served. What is the primary source of information that should be considered to modify the service environment to ensure visual affirmation in the area?

2. A healthcare facility, serving a significant number of patients from Jamaica, has an opening to recruit several new board members. The recruitment committee of the board decides that since they already have two African Americans on the board, out of a total of 15 members, more Jamaican members are not necessary. What is your view of that decision?

3. A number of incidents have occurred at a public health entity during which community members have complained of cultural bias. The public health official in charge of the facility recommends cultural competence training through the hiring of a consultant. However, there is concern that there would not be sufficient return on investment for the endeavor. Is this an accurate view? Explain.

4. The chief financial officer (CFO) of a healthcare organization expresses reservation regarding a department's request to purchase Native American artwork to hang on the walls of one of their sites that serves a Native American community in the nearby vicinity. The CFO expresses that such expenditure is frivolous and that the site is not a museum but a healthcare facility. The department director proceeds to show the CFO the demographic data of the customers served at the site, identifying them as primarily Native American (a specific local tribe), and explains that the current artwork reflects images of Caucasian people only. The director is concerned when her request remains an area of contention with the CFO and is ultimately denied. Is the director or the CFO right? Why?

5. The CEO advises the board of directors that it is necessary to revisit the mission statement of a healthcare organization to ensure that it reflects a commitment to cultural competence and diversity. The board members agree but decide that diversity and culture have the same meaning and that either one or the other should be included but not both. How should the CEO advise the board on this matter?

REFERENCES

Cohen, E., & Goode, T. D. (1999), revised by Toode, T. D., & Dunne, C. (2003). *Policy brief 1: Rationale for cultural competence in primary care.* Washington, DC: National Center for Cultural Competence, Georgetown Center for Child and Human Development.

Levinson, W., Roter D. L., Mullooly, J. P., Dull, V. T, & Frankel, R. M. (1997). Physician-patient communication: The relationship with malpractice claims among primary care physicians and surgeons. *Journal of the American Medical Association, 277,* 553–559.

Reynolds, D. (2004). Improving care and interactions with racially and ethnically diverse populations in healthcare organizations. *Journal of Healthcare Management, 49*(4), 237–246.

Robert Wood Johnson Foundation and Henry J. Kaiser Family Foundation. (1997). *Opening doors: Reducing sociocultural barriers to health care.* Retrieved March 7, 2008, from http://www.rwjf.org/pr/product.jsp?id=17978.

Smedley, B. D., Stith, A. Y., & Nelson, A. R. (Eds.). (2003). *Unequal treatment: Confronting racial and ethnic disparities in health care.* Washington, DC: The National Academies Press.

Suro, R. (2000, February). Beyond economics. *American Demographics.* Retrieved April 14, 2008, from http://findarticles.com/p/articles/mi_m4021/is_2000_Feb/ai_59834064/?tag=content;col1.

Thomas, D. (2004). Diversity as strategy. *Harvard Business Review, 1*(September), 98–108.

Waldren, C. A. (2004). Classical radiation biology dogma, bystander effects and paradigm shifts. *Human and Experimental Toxicology, 23,* 95–100.

Suggested Readings

Dana, R. H., & Allen, J. (2008). *Striving for cultural competence: Moving beyond potential and transforming the helping professions.* New York: Springer.

Henry J. Kaiser Foundation. (2003). *Compendium of cultural competence initiatives in health care.* Available at http://www.kff.org/uninsured/6067-index.cfm.

Jackson, P. (2008). *Developing a culturally competent workforce, part 2.* Available at http://www.hhnmag.com/hhnmag_app/jsp/articledisplay.jsp?dcrpath=HHNMAG/Article/data/06JUN2008/080624HHN_Online_Jackson&domain=HHNMAG.

Perez, M. A. (2008). *Cultural competence in health education and health promotion.* San Francisco: Jossey-Bass.

Yale Center for Public Health Preparedness. (2007). *Cultural and linguistic competence in public health preparedness.* Available at http://publichealth.yale.edu/ycphp/newsletters/2007newsletters/Cultural%20Competence.pdf.

Chapter 4

Understanding Cultural Nuances and Barriers to Cultural Appreciation

LEARNING OBJECTIVES

After reading this chapter, you should be able to:

- Discuss cultural nuances and their relevance to particular racial/ethnic groups.
- Explore cultural competence as a developmental process.
- Understand key social determinants and their relevance to cultural competence.
- Identify the concept of racial and ethnic disparities in health care.
- Discuss the need for diverse healthcare leadership and workforce in the provision of culturally competent care.
- Provide examples of treatment-seeking behaviors, expectations of care of specific racial/ethnic groups, and language differences/barriers.
- Describe linguistic competence within the context of cultural competence.

┌─ **KEY TERMS** ─────────────────────────────

Cultural nuances   Diversity
Linguistic competence   Stereotypes
Health disparity

INTRODUCTION

Within the context of various racial and ethnic groups, based on nationality, environment, culture, and other factors, there are specific cultural nuances, treatment-seeking behaviors, expectations of care, and language differences/barriers.

This chapter will explore the significance of understanding such differences and provide specific examples of each. The primary focus will be to explain how lack of diversity in healthcare leadership and workforce impacts the quality of care provided to patients and customers. The impact of the lack of culturally competent care will be highlighted linking health disparities to this problem.

CULTURAL NUANCES

A key aspect of cultural competence is recognizing **cultural nuances**, which are the subtle differences between particular cultures. Subtleties of individual cultures define a people's view of themselves and the perception of the world around them. By understanding these nuances, better interaction can be achieved in terms of culture and communication. For example, a cultural nuance specific to the Japanese population is the removal of one's shoes upon entering a home. This is a very strict requirement among many Japanese people, requiring the use of provided slippers prior to walking on the floors of their homes. Nonadherence to this requirement is considered rude, inappropriate, and unhygienic. As another example, in certain sects of the Muslim community, women are mostly covered and can only reveal certain body parts, usually their faces (in some instances, limited to their eyes, hands, and feet), when in public in an effort to maintain modesty, respect, and privacy for the women per their religious scripture, the Koran. Consequently, when a Muslim woman is cared for by a male physician, it is often required that a female relative be present for any examination of the patient. The best approach is for the woman to be seen by a female practitioner to avoid violation of the modesty requirement (Hollins, 2006). This cultural nuance requires sensitivity, understanding, and adherence to the requirement in order to maintain Muslim patients/clients/customers who are women and ensure respect and dignity for their culture. As a final example, people from Spain find stretching and yawning to be very bad manners and in poor taste. They are also very casual about keeping appointments (Graff, 2001). Keeping this in mind is important so as not to insult them by yawning or stretching in their presence or being overly upset if they miss an appointment but rather explaining the impact of their doing so in terms of scheduling. Awareness of cultural nuances over a broad base of cultures, races, and ethnicities will optimize the provision of services for individuals.

CULTURAL COMPETENCE AS A DEVELOPMENTAL PROCESS

In addition to optimizing the provision of services, cultural competence is a developmental process that evolves over an extended period of time, for both individuals and organizations, at various levels of awareness, knowledge, and skills along the cultural competence continuum (Cross, Bazron, Dennis, & Isaacs, 1989). This continuum, which will be discussed in detail in the next chapter, consists of six components or levels enabling individuals and organizations to determine their cultural competence status. Furthermore, cultural competence initiatives may help control cost by making care more efficient and effective (Betancourt, Green, Carrillo, & Park, 2005). The development and implementation of a robust cultural competence plan by health service organizations and public health entities must be a key strategy for success. The aim of such a plan should be to change from a one-size-fits-all system to one that is responsive to diverse populations. This requires diversity among board members, staff, and providers; enhanced data collection capacities; effective interpretation and translation services; and cultural competence education. It also requires that the organizations recognize and address their needs through both internal and external assessment processes. These processes should include consideration of the factors that currently define the delivery of health care in the United States, along with the compelling need for cultural competence to be incorporated into organizational policy. Some reasons that cultural competence is necessary include the changing demographics of the population; the need to eliminate disparities in the health status of people of diverse racial, ethnic, and cultural backgrounds; the improvement of the quality of services and health outcomes; compliance with legislative, regulatory, and accreditation mandates; strategies to gain market share; and strategies to decrease potential liability and/or malpractice claims (Cohen & Goode, 1999). Lack of awareness of differences, such as the cultural nuances described earlier (and additional insight in terms of health-seeking behaviors, expectations of care of specific racial/ethnic groups, cultural values and beliefs, and so on), and failure to provide translation and interpretation services may result in a lack of understanding and, subsequently, in breaches of professional standards of care or the presumption of negligence.

LINGUISTIC COMPETENCE

In addition to the previous definition provided in Chapter 2, another definition of **linguistic competence** is the ability to communicate effectively and accurately with individuals whose primary language is not English. Understanding of culture and respect for differences will allow healthcare managers to make more appropriate planning and intervention decisions. Patient satisfaction is reliant on an organization's ability to communicate and understand the cultural factors that affect health behavior (Betancourt et al., 2005). It is also important to take linguistic factors into consideration because language barriers can adversely affect the delivery of healthcare services in communities. Patients/clients/customers who are not proficient in English will often enter a healthcare facility or receive public health information and have no idea how to proceed because they cannot understand what is said to them, read the signage, or understand written materials provided to them. This can cause fear, apprehension, and miscommunication and impact treatment-seeking behaviors, compliance regarding instructions provided to them, treatment follow-up, and adherence to medication requirements. For example, in many states in the United States, disaster preparedness is critical. Public health organizations will often provide information on how to prepare for a disaster. If the literature, public service announcements, and other materials are only in English, individuals who are monolingual Creole or Spanish, for example, will be without insight if a disaster impacts their Haitian or Spanish-speaking (e.g., Cuban, Dominican, Costa Rican, and so on) communities

Furthermore, as stated by LaVeist (2002) in regard to the Hispanic population and language barriers:

> Previous studies have shown that Hispanic patients have lower health care use than white patients, including fewer physician visits and lower use of outpatient mental health, mammography, and influenza vaccinations. Our findings based on insured, non-elderly adults suggest that the Hispanic disparity in use is largely confined to Spanish-speaking Hispanic patients. These results are consistent with previous studies suggesting that lack of English fluency is associated with reduced health care use. Our study adds to this growing literature by showing that language fluency (or closely associated factors, such as acculturation) is the primary contributor to ethnic disparities in access to studied types of care among insured, non-elderly Hispanic adults. (p. 2005)

HEALTH DISPARITY

Thus far, the 21st century has been a period of ever-growing globalization, resulting in multiculturalism in the United States and elsewhere. The United States is considered a world leader in terms of medical technology. Nevertheless, equity does not exist in terms of the provision of health care because it is not distributed evenly throughout the US population. Although racial and ethnic minorities are fast-growing groups that will have greater numbers than the current majority, the White population, in coming years, a grim picture is provided by health statistics in terms of the health status of some minority groups compared with the mainstream population.

Health disparity is often referred to as healthcare inequality or gaps in the quality of health and health care across racial, ethnic, and socioeconomic groups. The Health Resources and Services Administration defines health disparity as "population-specific differences in the presence of disease, health outcomes or access to health care" (Carter-Pokras & Baquet, 2002, p. 430). The focus here is disparities pertaining to the quality of care that different ethnic and racial groups receive. Reasons for disparities in terms of access to health care, specifically, are attributed to many causes, such as low socioeconomic status, lack of insurance coverage, lack of a regular source of care, legal barriers, structural barriers, limits in terms of the healthcare financing system, scarcity of providers, linguistic barriers, lack of health literacy among certain groups and communities, cultural barriers, and lack of diversity in the healthcare workforce. Other factors are education, segregation, and immigration status (Kosoko-Lasaki, Cook, & O'Brien, 2009). Education is significant because there is a correlation between health outcomes and years in school. There is no doubt that education impacts employment, social status, and other factors. However, in American society, education alone may not be sufficient to explain difference in health outcomes because African Americans with high education levels (college) have poorer health outcomes. Differences in health outcomes may have more to do with exposure to positive or negative healthcare practices generationally; for example, African Americans are descendants of slaves and thus may have inherited the dietary preferences of slaves that have been passed on from one generation to the next, including highly seasoned and fried foods and other preparation methods that are less healthy than the foods and methods of other groups. Research was conducted in St. Louis, Missouri, in which the eating habits of the early African Americans were explored. The following was determined, as indicated in Kosoko-Lasaki et al.:

> During slavery they subsisted on "scraps" from the master's table, second-line (imperfect) crops, and pork. Organ meats such as brains or liver, fried foods, highly salted vegetables (greens) and unusual animal parts generally discarded by the master were prepared to ingenious fashions to add flavor. Cattle and beef were usually consumed by whites. Pig snoots, pig feet, brains, chitterlings, and tripe became the cuisine of the African American culture. (p. 335)

African Americans also live largely in poorer socioeconomic conditions and are more apt to be first-generation college students and may have issues associated with lack of cultural competence when seeking health care. As pointed out by LaVeist (2002):

> . . . that these disparities exist in some areas . . . suggests that the cost of care is an important consideration in clinical decisions for ethnic

> minority groups. Study findings that suggest the disparity is reduced for privately insured patients may also be an indication of payment-conscious clinical decisions. (p. 184)

Again, the less-than-positive health outcomes for African Americans are in part a result of eating patterns and culture; Kosoko-Lasaki et al. (2009) discuss these patterns and their cultural significance:

> A very interesting article from the 2001 *Journal of Archaeology*, entitled "Ham Hocks on Your Cornflakes" examined the role of food in the African American Identity. Excavations in Annapolis, Maryland, and 13 other sites in the Chesapeake region were explored. Findings were consistent; food remains showed a definite pattern. Pork was much more commonly consumed than beef, and shallow water fish not typically purchased from markets where whites typically shopped predominated. Apparently, by the late 19th century as whites turned to beef, blacks did not. . . . For many people, eating particular foods serves not only as a fulfilling experience, but also a liberating one—an added way of making some kind of declaration. Consumption then is at the same time a form of self-identification and communication. Blacks living under the oppression of slavery, with very few options, gathered at the end of the day for a communal meal with friends and family They most likely found spiritual strength and regeneration through eating and camaraderie. This experience over generations became a part of the culture. (p. 335)

Hence, although education provides one with more information and insight into what it takes to be healthy, it may not be enough to override social factors and long-term exposure to cultural norms.

Segregation is also a factor in health disparity because, although the United States is extremely diverse, groups of people are largely segregated by race. According to Massey and Denton (1994), affluent Black people earning $50,000 or more are more segregated than Hispanic/Latino or Asian people earning less than $15,000 per year. This may largely be due to the fact that many Hispanic/Latino people classify themselves as White Hispanic/Latino because Hispanic/Latino is not a race but an ethnicity and, therefore, are more apt to live among White people and function as White Hispanics/Latinos. Members of various Asian groups tend to assimilate more rapidly in the United States than other racial groups and, as a consequence, may not segregate to the same degree as African Americans. In addition, Asian and White Hispanic people have better access to credit and mortgage loans in the United States due to less discrimination directed toward them compared with Black people. Consequently, this also leads to less segregation and acquisition of homes in largely White communities where there is greater access to healthcare and other health-related services.

Immigration is another significant factor in terms of health disparities primarily because many immigrant populations do not have access to health care. Although community health centers in the United States are available to serve undocumented persons, the problem is that most people, including immigrant and nonimmigrant groups, are not aware of these facilities and the fact that people can be seen at these facilities regardless of their ability to pay or their immigration status. Hence, many immigrants have poorer health because they will seek care in emergency rooms or not seek care at all because they believe they will be asked for documentation that may lead to their deportation. The health disparities framework in Table 4-1 provides further insight. Some of the key disparities in terms of the various racial/ethnic groups are listed in Table 4-2.

Table 4-1 Health Disparities Framework

Health—Before Care	Access to Care	Healthcare Delivery
Income levels, poverty, and other social conditions	Financial resources	Insurance coverage and type
Safety and adequacy of housing	Availability and proximity of providers	Cultural competency levels
Employment status and type of employment	Access to transportation	Patient–provider communications
Education levels	Insurance coverage	Provider discrimination or bias
Lifestyle choices—diet, exercise, tobacco, and alcohol use	Regular source of care	Differential propensities for certain diseases by racial/ethnic populations
Environmental conditions—air and water quality, pesticide exposure, green space	Language barriers	Patient preferences and adherence to treatment plans
	Legal barriers (e.g., eligibility restrictions, illegal immigrants)	Diversity of the healthcare workforce
	Prior experience with the healthcare system	Appropriateness of care
	Cultural preferences—care-seeking behaviors	Effectiveness of care
	Health literacy levels	Language barriers
	Diversity of the healthcare workforce	

Source: Courtesy of Health Policy Institute of Ohio. (2004, September). *Understanding health disparities.*

Table 4-2 A Glimpse of Health Disparities

African Americans[a]	Hispanic Americans[a]	American Indians/ Alaska Natives	Asian and Pacific Islanders[b]
• More likely to develop cancer than persons of any other racial or ethnic group. • Have the highest cancer death rate than any other racial or ethnic group. • Around 40% of men and women have some form of heart disease, compared to 30% of White men and 24% of White women, and are 29% more likely to die from the disease than Whites. • Twice as likely to have diabetes as Whites. • In 2001, the infant mortality rate was more than twice the rate for White infants (13.3 deaths per 1000 for African Americans vs 5.7 for Whites).	• Die from heart disease at a lesser rate than Whites, but Mexican American women are diagnosed with the condition more frequently than White females. • In men, Mexican Americans have a higher prevalence of overweight and obesity than non-Hispanic men. • Within the Puerto Rican subgroup, the rate of infant deaths from sudden infant death syndrome (SIDS) is 1.5 times higher than Whites.	• The incidence of diabetes is more than twice that of Whites.[a] • The death rate is 70% higher than in Whites.[a] • Among youth aged 10–19 years, American Indians have the highest prevalence of type 2 diabetes of any racial/ethnic group.[c] • Suicide rates among American Indians/Alaska Natives aged 15–34 years are more than 2 times higher than the national average for that age group.[c]	• In 2006, Asian Americans were 1.2 times more likely to have hepatitis B than Whites. • Asian/Pacific Islander men are twice as likely to die from stomach cancer compared to the non-Hispanic White population, and Asian/Pacific Islander women are 2.6 times as likely to die from the same disease. • In Hawaii, native Hawaiians have more than twice the rate of diabetes as Whites.

[a] Data from Department of Health and Human Services (DHHS). (2007). *Fact sheet: Minority health disparities at a glance*. Retrieved November 16, 2009, from http://www.omhrc.gov/templates/contentaspx?ID=2139.

[b] Data from The Office of Minority Health. (2009). *Asian American profile*. Retrieved November 16, 2009, from http://www.omhrc.gov/templates/content.aspx?ID=3005.

[c] Data from Centers for Disease Control and Prevention. (2009). *Health disparities and ethnic minority youth*. Retrieved November 16, 2009, from http://www.cdc.gov/Features/HealthDisparities/.

Cultural competence is "evolving from a marginal to a mainstream health care policy issue and as a potential strategy to improve quality and address disparities" (Curtis, Dreachslin, & Sinioris, 2007). For healthcare organizations, cultural competence strategy and training must be responsive to aims developed toward improving quality of care. Some of these aims have been developed by the Institute of Medicine, for example, and include safe, effective, patient-centered, timely, efficient, and equitable care. Furthermore, responsiveness to the national standards for Culturally and Linguistically Appropriate Services in Health Care, set forth by the US Department of Health and Human Services Office of Minority Health, will also help in relieving health disparities (Curtis et al.). A successful example of a culturally competent system of care is described in the Child and Adolescent Service System Program (CASSP), where the care and services focus on the family as the primary support and community-based approaches as part of informal support systems (e.g., churches, neighborhoods, healers). This also entails introducing choice in service, incorporation of cultural knowledge into practice and policy making, less restrictive alternatives, and adequate cross-cultural communication to achieve goals (Cross et al., 1989).

DIVERSE HEALTHCARE LEADERSHIP

Diversity includes all of the distinctions and differences between people. Aspects of diversity include race, gender, age, physical appearance, nationality, cultural heritage, life experience, mental and physical differences, economic status, religion, language, marital status, educational level, sexual orientation, and so on. Cultural competence in health care cannot be achieved without diversity and strong leadership within healthcare organizations. Assessment must take place over time to ensure that there is an understanding of demographic changes. The board of directors of healthcare organizations should ideally be a representative microcosm of the communities served by health service organizations. Consequently, boards should strive to choose leaders, namely the president/chief executive officer (CEO)/administrator, of institutions who value diversity. Furthermore, human resources and education staff should be leaders in development of criteria for the hiring of diverse staff and training of employees at all levels to ensure an optimum level of cultural competence. Within healthcare organizations, it is not only processes that must be adapted to embrace cultural diversity and cultural competence, but also the people who serve as frontline staff. It cannot be expected that every individual within an organization will have insight into every culture because there are so many cultures and also many differences within cultures. Hence, first and foremost, individuals in an organization should acknowledge that patients/clients/customers from various cultures will often have different values and customs from their own culture. Healthcare institutions and public health entities must ensure that resources are in place to meet the varying needs of their patients/clients/customers.

CULTURE, RACE, AND ETHNICITY AS A FACTOR IN THE DOCTOR–PATIENT RELATIONSHIP

The idea of physician bias was popularized in a report published by the Institute of Medicine in 2003 entitled *Unequal Treatment: Confronting Racial and Ethnic Disparities in Health Care*. This report concluded that an important dynamic in race-related treatment difference was bias, prejudice, and discrimination within the doctor–patient relationship. It is also believed that the patient–doctor relationship has an important impact on disparities in medical care (Street, 2008). Although some research has supported the idea that race, ethnicity, and culture play a crucial role in the doctor–patient relationship, others have argued that socioeconomic status is also a critical factor (LaVeist, 2002). It is important for health administrators to be aware of these perspectives to ensure that such insight is provided in terms of cultural competence training for providers and staff.

Specifically, race and ethnicity have been cited as important cultural barriers in patient–doctor communication, and yet cross-cultural factors have been relatively unexplored (LaVeist, 2002). Research has shown that racial and ethnic differences between doctor and patient not only influence physician communications but also decision making. However, these studies also show an enhancement of communication and decision making when the doctor and patient are of the same race or culture (LaVeist). This indicates that racial and cultural differences may be significant barriers to partnership and effective communication. A number of factors may account for this barrier in communication. One of these factors may be "unintentionally incorporated racial biases" (LaVeist), which is the idea that unconscious racial stereotypes may have been integrated into patients' symptoms and predictions of patients' behaviors and thus have become part of medical decision making.

The term stereotype was coined in 1978 during the onset of the modern industrial age. The image-setting process was called stereotyping, and over time, the word stereotype came to apply to the fixing of intellectual, as opposed to printed, images (Fuligni, 2007). Defining the term stereotype today, in terms of people, is complex. There are hundreds of possible definitions, even though they are all based on the idea that stereotypes are knowledge structures that serve as mental "pictures" of the group in question. With some exceptions, the general consensus is that stereotypes represent the traits viewed as characteristics of social groups or of individual members of those groups, particularly those characteristics that differentiate groups from each other (Wheeler, Jarvis, & Petty, 2001). In short, **stereotypes** are exaggerated beliefs or fixed ideas about a person, and the term is taught within the context of a particular example that expresses how this process can impact the provision of services to an individual. However, the tendency to oversimplify the definition has led to abandoning some of the presumed characteristics of stereotyping that were so critical to its early conceptualization as a result of inaccuracy, negativity, and overgeneralization. Stereotypes are usually negative, inaccurate, and unfair; otherwise, they would simply be part of the broad study of human perception (Lee, Jussim, & McCauley, 1995). In terms of cultural competence, stereotypes matter because they influence judgment and behavior. Social categorization often occurs as a consequence of stereotyping, which usually transpires upon first meeting another person, without any real intention or awareness on the part of the person who is doing the categorizing (Nelson, 2009).

Another cause of barriers between patients and providers may be the lack of understanding of the patients' ethnic and cultural models or attributions of symptoms. This lack of understanding could lead to the patient being misdiagnosed. The final cause of barriers suggested by LaVeist (2002) is that physicians and patients have different expectations of the visits or physicians are unaware of patients' expectations of visits. Other factors that may contribute to communication barriers between doctors and patients are language barriers, low health literacy, and educational status.

Essentially, communication barriers between physicians and patients, no matter the cause, in terms of race, culture, and ethnicity contribute to ongoing health disparities. When a doctor and patient are of the same race and culture, they are likely to have more in common than if they are of different races. Physicians and patients of the same race or ethnic group are more likely to share cultural beliefs, values, and experiences. This enables more effective communication because the individuals may be more comfortable with each other. Physicians have indicated that when their patients are from similar backgrounds, empathy is present automatically and that when treating patients that have different racial and cultural backgrounds from their own, there are fewer shared experiences (Chen, 2008).

TREATMENT-SEEKING BEHAVIORS

Based on race, culture, and ethnicity, particular treatment-seeking behaviors exist that, on a generalized basis, need to be taken into consideration. As examples, the cultures of Mexican, Haitian, Native American, and Southern Black people and their definitions of health and illness will be explored. One should not view the perspectives offered here as the case for all members of these groups because that would lead to stereotyping. However, based

Table 4-3 Selected Behaviors/Perspectives of Various Groups That May Impact Treatment-Seeking Behaviors

Culture	Behaviors/Perspectives
Mexicans	• Health is a gift from God and a reward for good behavior.
	• Health results from maintaining balance in the universe between "hot" and "cold" forces. Illness in an individual body is considered a punishment meted out for some wrong doing.
Haitians	• Health is a state of harmony with nature. Illness is a state of disharmony and is also caused by movement of blood, problems with gas, imbalance between "hot" and "cold" forces, and voodoo or a spell placed on a person. To maintain health, the spirit and body must be linked together by the soul.
	• May not feel comfortable discussing their spirit and soul with a medical practitioner for fear that their explanation may be misunderstood.
Native Americans	• Health is a state of total harmony with nature; human beings have an intimate relationship with nature.
	• Illness is considered a price paid for something that happened in the past or that will happen in the future. Illness may also be due to evil spirits.
Southern Blacks	• May feel that their illness is due to sin or evil.
	• May feel that an illness such as a cold is due to weather rather than a microbiologic factor (e.g., going out in cold weather will cause one to catch a cold).

Source: Data from Giger, J. N., & Davidhizar, R. E. (1991). *Transcultural nursing, assessment and intervention*. St. Louis, MO: Mosby Year Book.

on research pertaining to the groups, some commonalities have surfaced among people within the same groups (Table 4-3).

Mexican people, in general, view health as a gift from God and a reward for good behavior. Health results from maintaining balance in the universe between "hot" and "cold" forces. Illness in an individual's body is considered a punishment meted out for some wrongdoing. Haitian people, on the other hand, view health as a state of harmony with nature and illness as a state of disharmony. To maintain health, the spirit and the body must be linked together by the soul. Illness is caused by movement of blood, problems with gas imbalance between "hot" and "cold" forces, and voodoo or a spell placed on a person. Additionally, although there are many different groups/tribes with different cultural norms, Native American people generally believe that health is a state of total harmony with nature and that human beings have an intimate relationship with nature. Illness is considered a price being paid for something that happened in the past or that will happen in the future. Some

Native Americans believe that illness may also be due to evil spirits. Southern Black people may feel that their illness is due to sin or evil. They may also feel that their illnesses are a result of weather rather than microbiologic factors (Giger & Davidhizar, 1991); for example, they might believe that if one goes outside in cold weather, he or she will catch a cold as a result, rather than the cold being a result of a microbiologic (bacterial or viral) cause.

As a consequence of these beliefs, people from different cultures may have different treatment-seeking behaviors. Specifically, southern Black people may not seek care if they feel that their illnesses are due to sin or evil, and they may not want to reveal the supposed sin to healthcare practitioners. Furthermore, Haitians may not feel comfortable discussing their spirit and soul with a medical practitioner for fear that their explanation will be misunderstood. Hence, these examples illustrate how cultural perspectives may affect treatment-seeking behaviors within the context of cultural competence. Health service administrators and public health officials should ensure that all staff and providers are trained in the cultures of the specific groups served by their organization based on demographic data. This will build trust with patients.

CONCLUSIONS

A number of factors must be taken into consideration when trying to understand cultural nuances and barriers to cultural understanding. It is very difficult for health service administrators and public health practitioners to ensure optimal services without considering the needs of various racial and ethnic groups and making sure that providers and staff have an understanding of cultural nuances, cultural beliefs and values, and treatment-seeking behaviors and their relevance. Diversity in healthcare leadership and workforce provides a better basis for moving in the direction of understanding because it sets the tone for overcoming barriers to care among racial and ethnic minorities. Diversification alone, however, is insufficient. Making sure that specific skills pertaining to cultural and linguistic competence are provided at every level of health service and public health organizations is paramount, with the goal being to offer top-notch services leading to the elimination of racial and ethnic health disparities.

CHAPTER SUMMARY

Cultural competence is a developmental process that takes place over time. It requires an understanding of key social determinants, namely socioeconomic status and its impact on health disparities from a racial and ethnic vantage point. Furthermore, treatment-seeking behaviors, based on diversity and cultural nuances specific to cultural and ethnic groups, must be understood. Linguistic competence is also a critical factor because language can serve as a barrier and impact treatment-seeking behaviors, leading to health disparities. Such language barriers may also impact expectations of care for individuals seeking optimal health care. Linguistic competence is a key component of cultural competency because language is also a part of culture, and it is the responsibility of the health service organization and public health practitioners to meet the needs of their customers on every level.

CHAPTER PROBLEMS

1. A Haitian woman arrives at a healthcare facility in pain and in need of desperate care. She tries to explain that a spell has been placed on her and she needs an immediate remedy. She is monolingual Creole speaking. What steps should be taken at the healthcare facility to handle her situation?

2. There is a distinct health disparity between Blacks and Whites in the United States. What are some issues that may serve as contributing factors to the problem?

3. Health service administrators often acknowledge the need for cultural competence training within their organization as well as a diverse staff. Describe the steps that they may need to be taken to ensure a diverse staff and the necessary training.

4. Socioeconomic status is often described as a determinant of health and a contributing factor relevant to racial health disparities. Explain why this is so.

5. At a monthly board meeting, a board member expresses that the health center that he serves is in the United States and that the predominant language spoken in the United States is English. Therefore, he sees no need for linguistic competence to be an aspect of concern for the organization because patients who seek care need to learn to speak English. What might the CEO say to the board member when she emphasizes the need for a fundraiser to acquire funds to implement costly translation and interpretation services throughout the healthcare facility, necessitating board participation?

REFERENCES

Betancourt, J., Green, A., Carrillo, M., & Park, E. (2005). Cultural competence and health care disparities: Key perspectives and trends. *Health Affairs, 24*(2), 502–505.

Carter-Pokras, O., & Baquet, C. (2002). What is a health disparity? *Public Health Reports, 117,* 426–434.

Chen, P. (2008, November 14). Confronting the racial barriers between doctors and patients. *The New York Times.*

Cohen, E., & Goode, T. D. (1999), revised by Goode, T. D., & Dunne, C. (2003). *Policy brief 1: Rationale for cultural competence in primary care.* Washington, DC: National Center for Cultural Competence, Georgetown Center for Child and Human Development.

Cross, T., Bazron, B., Dennis, K., & Isaacs, M. (1989). *Towards a culturally competent system of care* (Vol. 1). Washington, DC: Georgetown University Child Development Center, CASSP Technical Assistance Center.

Curtis, E. F., Dreachslin, J. L., & Sinioris, M. (2007). Diversity and cultural competence training in health care organizations: Hallmarks of success. *The Health Care Manager, 26*(3), 255–262.

Fuligni, A. (2007). *Contesting stereotypes and creating identities: Social categories, social identities and educational participation.* New York: Russell Sage Foundation.

Giger, J. N., & Davidhizar, R. E. (1991). *Transcultural nursing, assessment and intervention.* St. Louis, MO: Mosby Year Book.

Graff, M. L. (2001). *Culture shock! A guide to customs and etiquette: Spain.* Portland, OR: Graphic Arts Center Publishing Company.

Hollins, S. (2006). *Religions, culture and healthcare: A practical handbook for use in healthcare environments.* Oxford, UK: Radcliffe Publishing.

Institute of Medicine. (2003). *Unequal treatment: Confronting racial and ethnic disparities in health care.* Retrieved November 15, 2009, from http://www.iom .edu/en/Reports/2003/Unequal-Treatment-Confronting-Racial-and-Ethnic-Disparities-in-Health-Care.aspx.

Kosoko-Lasaki, S., Cook, C., & O'Brien, R. (2009). *Cultural proficiency in addressing health disparities.* Sudbury, MA: Jones and Bartlett Publishers.

LaVeist, T. (2002). *Race, ethnicity and health: A public health reader.* San Francisco: John Wiley & Sons.

Lee, Y., Jussim, L., & McCauley, C. (1995). *Stereotype accuracy.* Washington, DC: American Psychological Association.

Massey, D. S., & Denton, N. A. (1994). *American apartheid: Segregation and the making of the underclass.* Boston: Harvard University Press.

Nelson, T. (2009). *Handbook of prejudice, stereotyping and discrimination.* New York: Psychology Press.

Street, R. (2008). Understanding concordance in patient-physician relationships. *Annals of Family Medicine, 6*(3), 198–205.

Wheeler, S. C., Jarvis, B. G. & Petty, R. E. (2001). The effects of sterotype activiation on behavior: A review of possible racial stereotypes. *Journal of Experimental Social Psychology, 37*, 173–180.

SUGGESTED READINGS

Cross, T. L. (1995). Understanding family resiliency from a relational world view. In H. I. McCubbin, E. A. Thompson, A. I. Thompson, & J. E. Fromer (Eds.), *Resiliency in ethnic minority families. Volume I: Native and immigrant American families.* Madison, WI: University of Wisconsin System.

Fadiman, A. (1997). *The spirit catches you and you fall down*. New York: Farrar, Strauss and Giroux.

Levy, D. (1985). White doctors and black patients: Influence of race on the doctor-patient relationship. *Pediatrics, 75*, 639–643.

Mayberry, R. M., Mili, F., & Ofili, E. (2002). Racial and ethnic differences in access to medical care. In T. LaVeist (Ed.), *Race, ethnicity and health: A public health reader* (p. 170). San Francisco: John Wiley & Sons.

Mensah, G., & Glover, M. J. (2007). Epidemiology of racial and ethnic disparities in health and healthcare. In R. A. Williams (Ed.), *Eliminating healthcare disparities in America: Beyond the IOM report*. Totowa, NJ: Humana Press.

Rubin, R., & Melnick, J. (2007). *Immigration and American popular culture*. New York: New York University Press.

Washington, H. (2006). *Medical apartheid: The dark history of medical experimentation on Black Americans from colonial times to the present*. New York: Doubleday.

The Cultural Competence Continuum

After reading this chapter, you should be able to:

- Explain the Cultural Competence Continuum and all of its components.
- Understand the parameters that differentiate cultures.
- Discuss the Cultural Competence Framework.
- Facilitate the Assumption Exercise.
- Define terms such as ethnocentric and all terms associated with the Cultural Competence Continuum.

KEY TERMS

Cultural awareness	Cultural incapacity
Cultural blindness	Cultural knowledge
Cultural competence	Cultural precompetence
Cultural desire	Cultural proficiency
Cultural destructiveness	Cultural skill
Cultural encounters	

INTRODUCTION

This chapter provides an overview of the Cultural Competence Continuum. Thus, the focus will be cultural destructiveness, cultural incapacity, cultural blindness, cultural precompetence, cultural competence, and cultural proficiency, which are all components of the continuum. A Cultural Competence Framework will also be explored, including cultural awareness, encounters, skills, and desires. Additionally, an exercise, called the Assumption Exercise, will be introduced that will enable exploration of cultural biases. This exercise is generally used for learning/training purposes within the context of cultural competence workshops. If assumptions are identified within the context of cultural competence training and workshops, it is possible to preclude misconceptions about patients/clients/customers that may lead to less than efficacious care. This exercise is also relevant for public health practitioners because public health is concerned with the broader population in terms of disease prevention, health promotion, community efforts, and so on and, thus, understanding of cultures is extremely important in the field.

CULTURAL COMPETENCE CONTINUUM

The Cultural Competence Continuum (Fig. 5-1) consists of six components or levels, with cultural destructiveness being the lowest level and cultural proficiency being the highest level and the ultimate goal to strive for (Cross, Bazron, Dennis, & Isaacs, 1989). Health service administrators and public health practitioners should become familiar with this continuum and its various components because it will help to ensure maximum cultural efficiency in serving diverse communities. This continuum enables an organization to determine its cultural competence status and to ensure that

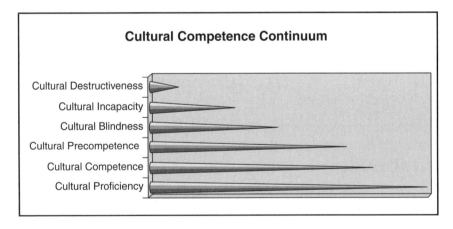

Figure 5-1 Cultural competence continuum.
Source: Data from Cross, T., Bazron, B., Dennis, K., & Isaacs, M. (1989). *Towards a culturally competent system of care* (Vol. 1). Washington, DC: Child and Adolescent Service System Program Technical Assistance Center, Center for Child and Mental Health Policy, Georgetown University Child Development Center.

the goal is to strive to be at the optimum level of the continuum (cultural proficiency) rather than at the bottom level (cultural destructiveness), where serious harm can take place, both intentionally and unintentionally.

Cultural Destructiveness

Cultural destructiveness refers to attitudes, policies, practices, and structures within a system or organization that are destructive to a cultural group (Cross et al., 1989). Often in a society or organization, certain practices or policies may be in place that are aimed at destroying a particular culture. For example, with the advent of chattel slavery in American society, when Africans were forcibly brought to the New World, all aspects of the slaves' African culture were destroyed; for example, they were not allowed to speak the languages of their native land; wear African attire; wear their intricate hairstyles; play their music, which consisted mainly of drumming and was often used as a communication mechanism; and practice their religions. Although this is an extreme example, it is specifically pertinent to the concept of cultural destructiveness. In a healthcare facility or in a public health setting, examples of cultural destructiveness would be requiring a Muslim woman to wear a short hospital gown with an opening in the back and disallowing her head covering in a hospital setting; these requirements run completely counter to her religious beliefs and codes. These examples may seem trivial to some people, but for the Muslim woman, it may prevent her from being able to receive care at the facility. Cultural destructiveness in health care and public health represents a complete lack of understanding and willingness to understand other cultures and involves setting up boundaries and requirements that force an individual or group of individuals to change in order to receive necessary services.

Cultural Incapacity

Cultural incapacity refers to the lack of capacity to respond effectively to culturally and linguistically diverse groups. Characteristics include, but are not limited to, institutional or systemic bias, practices that may result in discrimination in hiring and promotion, disproportionate allocation of resources that may benefit one cultural group over another, subtle messages that some cultural groups are neither valued nor welcome, and lower expectations for some cultural, ethnic, or racial groups (Cross et al., 1989). Examples include failure to provide interpreters for individuals who speak languages other than English and stating that in order to receive health services or to experience public health efforts, one must speak English.

Cultural Blindness

Cultural blindness refers to viewing all people the same, without taking into consideration that cultural differences matter. As a consequence of cultural blindness, little value is placed on training; there is limited diversity, if any, among personnel; and policies and personnel encourage assimilation and institutional attitudes that blame consumers for their circumstances (including families or individuals) if they believe that that they are not receiving optimal care based on cultural factors (Cross et al., 1989). A specific example would be a facility that has a predominantly mainstream staff when the majority of the individuals receiving services at the facility are from one or more minority groups and perhaps speak different languages and have varying dietary habits, religious practices, and so on. Failure to pay attention to and tailor services to meet these differences can be very problematic for healthcare and public health organizations.

Cultural Precompetence

Cultural precompetence is when a healthcare organization is aware of its strengths and areas for growth and there is a clear commitment to human and civil rights. Organizations at the cultural precompetence level have hiring practices that support a diverse workforce and a capacity to conduct needs assessments to determine where there are limitations. There is also a concerted effort to improve service delivery. However, generally, there is a tendency for token representation on governing boards and no clear plan for achieving organizational cultural competence and diversity. At this stage, there is an expressed recognition of the value of high-quality services, and there is a desire to support culturally and linguistically diverse populations (Cross et al., 1989). Although the beginnings of positive movement toward cultural competence are present, cultural precompetence is a very preliminary stage, and healthcare and public health organizations should make every effort to move beyond this stage. Initiative needs to be established to put plans in place to move the organization forward from a cultural competency, linguistic competency, and diversity standpoint.

Cultural Competence

Cultural competence, per the continuum, involves ensuring that the needs of diverse patients/clients/customers are met by health service and public health organizations based on the acquisition of specific skill sets, valuing diversity, and taking concrete steps to ensure efficacy in serving minority populations. The mission of health service and public health organizations should reflect the intention to adhere to cultural competence as well as specific policies and procedures relating to such a mission. This includes recruiting, hiring, and maintaining a diverse and culturally and linguistically competent workforce; dedicating resources for self-assessment and training regarding matters of cultural and linguistic competence; and the involvement of community participation at all levels (Cross et al., 1989). Furthermore, cultural competence entails, in general, the awareness and acceptance of difference, insight into one's own cultural values, understanding the dynamics of difference, development of cultural knowledge, and the ability to adapt practice skills to fit the cultural context of clients. Cultural competence goes beyond cultural awareness and sensitivity, emphasizing the idea of effectively operating in different cultural contexts (Cross et al., 1989). Furthermore, the notion of tolerance of diverse groups is not viewed as a favorable aspect of this component of the continuum because at this stage, there is clear understanding that all cultures must be valued and appreciated, not merely tolerated, with a clear goal toward meeting the needs of patients/clients/customers without judgment or criticism or imposing requirements that would be counter to specific cultures.

Cultural Proficiency

Cultural proficiency takes the process of cultural competence a step further by employing staff and consultants with cultural expertise, ensuring assessment and training efforts, and reviewing policies and procedures to ensure the inclusion of culturally competent language. At this level, active pursuit of resource development is maintained, and health service board members, executives, management, and staff advocate with and on behalf of populations who reflect the various cultures served by the organization to ensure maximum efficacy in meeting their needs (Cross et al., 1989). Additionally, resources are explored that can be used to take the healthcare or public health organization to the positive end of the continuum without hesitation or fiscal concerns because the benefits of doing so are understood. Although the term proficiency is used here, cultural proficiency is the highest level of the overall concept of cultural competence.

CULTURAL COMPETENCE FRAMEWORK

Per Campinha-Bacote (1999), cultural competence, beyond the continuum just described, is also divided into five interdependent constructs: cultural awareness, cultural knowledge, cultural skill, cultural encounters, and cultural desires.

> **Cultural awareness** is the ability of healthcare providers to appreciate and understand their clients' "values, beliefs, life ways, practices, and problem solving strategies" (Campinha-Bacote, 1999, p. 204). Self-awareness is also a vital part of this construct and allows healthcare providers to analyze their own beliefs to avoid bias and prejudice when working with clients.
>
> **Cultural knowledge** is the ability to have insight and knowledge about physical, physiologic, and biologic variations among groups, as well as knowledge about various cultures, to better understand clients.
>
> **Cultural skill** is the ability of healthcare providers to conduct an accurate and culturally competent history and physical examination.
>
> **Cultural encounters** is the ability of healthcare providers to competently work directly with clients of culturally diverse backgrounds. This is demonstrated by verbal and nonverbal messages by the healthcare provider and the client.
>
> **Cultural desire** is the ability of the healthcare provider, health service administrator, or public health practitioner to possess a drive to achieve cultural competence.

PARAMETERS THAT DIFFERENTIATE CULTURES

In considering the concept of cultural competence and implementing efforts to move to the most favorable end of the continuum, it is important to understand that there are many parameters that differentiate cultures. To illustrate this point, several of these parameters will be considered. The first considers views of time and space. For example, references have often been made to the notion of "colored people time," or CPT, or "Cuban time," which refers to the idea that people from African American and Cuban groups are often late for scheduled events, including healthcare appointments. Clearly, this is a stereotypical viewpoint, but it may represent, in social settings in particular, a more relaxed world view about time, amongst these groups compared with certain segments of mainstream Western culture. Being prompt is generally valued, but a relaxed attitude regarding time is often found in African, Caribbean, Latin, and Native American people and other cultures outside of the mainstream group in the United States. The problem occurs when it is presumed that members of these groups are incapable of being on time. This is inaccurate and a pejorative understanding of the concept, lending to a stereotypical and thus negative view of a behavior that is loosely associated with culture.

As another example, physical space between people is considered differently among cultures. In some societies, particularly among mainstream Americans, there is a perspective that there is an invisible space around individuals in which one should not enter. Therefore, it is expected that one person will not enter another person's "personal space" without permission because intimacy may be implied by doing so. In some cultures, however, people do not necessarily adhere to such space barriers and will speak to each other in very close proximity or find themselves in another person's "personal space" without a problem ensuing, even when intimacy is not involved. This close proximal space boundary can be found, for example, among people living in India and also Indians who have immigrated to America. Factors that have been speculated to contribute to this comfort with close contact include poverty and resulting overcrowded living environments, and differing views concerning proximal contact; regardless, culturally, it is more acceptable among many Indian people to be close in proximity or in another person's "personal space" than among mainstream Americans. Again, one has to be careful not to stereotype any particular group regarding space issues. Taking some time to understand cultural factors about the society from where people come (national origin), even though they are now residing in the United States, will give insight into cultural norms that may be different from those of the American mainstream.

Another parameter that should be considered from a cultural vantage point is that of gender roles. Clearly, there are a number of social constructs that determine the roles of men and women in various cultures, but the key is to understand that there are differences, based on culture, that need to be considered in terms of healthcare provision and public health practices. For example, in Islamic culture, modesty is valued, and it may be necessary to ensure that same-sex providers are used in the provision of care, particularly for women. A woman may need to be seen by a female provider, and a man may need to be seen by a male provider. Violation of this requirement may be deemed highly insensitive and may preclude further visits to a given healthcare facility or public health entity if the request for such modesty is not honored. Another example of a gender-specific situation involves the Hispanic culture; although the culture varies based on nationality and other factors within this ethnic group, generally, males are dominant. Often, an Hispanic woman will defer decision making about her health care to her husband or another male figure in the family.

Essentially, the key is to understand, as explained by Veneta Masson, RN (2005), that the entire point in regard to the provision of health care and culture is "to get to know the patient, his or her family, his or her living situation and the community over time and to allow yourself to be known."

Successful healthcare organizations are those that promote an environment in which the notion of looking into the faces of their charges (as opposed to serving them without making eye contact or making an effort to know them on a human level) and making sure that all who are involved in ensuring optimal care are consciously and subconsciously affirming that notion. It is important to ask key questions in the context of serving patients/clients/customers seeking health care to be sure that what they value, in terms of cultural requirements, are considered carefully. Furthermore, it is extremely important to know about different cultures, beliefs, attitudes, and values and to understand those cultures that are typically encountered by a given healthcare organization or public health facility. It is impossible to know everything about a culture, but if healthcare administrators and public health practitioners ensure that all staff, providers, and other employees are diverse and knowledgeable and are aware of certain parameters of culture, such as time and space, gender differences, rituals, beliefs about health, and other key aspects of culture, better provision of service will be the outcome. Although variations within cultural groups and among individuals exist, the more cultural knowledge that is acquired, the better equipped providers will be to ensure cultural competence.

THE ASSUMPTION EXERCISE

In an effort to begin the process of determining the level of cultural competence that is present at a healthcare organization or public health facility, various forms of assessment may be necessary. The process of assessment is discussed in depth in Chapter 7. However, a preliminary step is to explore the notion of assumptions that people may tend to make about others based on first impressions. The Assumption Exercise is useful and entails acquiring at least five pictures of individuals who represent a visual stereotypical image but differ from that image completely in terms of their profession or other characteristics. For example, during the Assumption Exercise, a picture is shown of an African American young man, originally born in Jamaica and now residing in the United States, who has the following appearance: long thick dreadlocks, skin of a very dark hue, and wearing baggy, loosely fitting jeans, a baseball cap, and oversized tee shirt. Participants are then asked to write down their first response to the image. Most who observe the photograph will often assume that the young man is a rap artist or musician or will sometimes indicate nefarious behavior, such as being a member of a gang or drug dealer, based on stereotypical characterizations of Black men who do not look like mainstream Americans. However, in reality, the young man in the picture is a Fulbright Scholar, holds a PhD, and is a motivational speaker, educational consultant, and instructional strategist. He also speaks seven languages, including Korean, learned during his visiting professorship at a university in South Korea; plays classical piano; and sings arias. Hence, incorrect assumptions are often made when one "judges a book by its cover."

The Assumption Exercise is an important exercise and often serves as a precursor to subsequent cultural competence assessment. A series of photos can be shown of various individuals who may appear to fit stereotypes but have characteristics that are counter to expected first impressions. Participants should write down their immediate response to each image shown; responses should be anonymous and reviewed by the facilitator. Next, the following questions should be asked of the participants: Did you make assumptions about the individuals in the pictures? Were your assumptions negative or positive? Why?

Often, this brief but powerful exercise will open the eyes of participants to help them understand that often judgments are made about individuals without knowing anything about them. The judgments are usually based on unfounded assumptions and a lack of understanding of one's cultural variations. In the earlier example, judging the African American man negatively based on his appearance and stereotypes may lead to hostility when providing health care or public health services or engender a range of concerns from fear to animosity. When performed effectively, this exercise can initiate dialogue concerning the issue of cultural competence, the need for it, and the various levels associated with it; these issues can be discussed in an environment of trust and comfort and lead to serious discourse about the importance of understanding, valuing, and appreciating other cultures. It is important for health service administrators and public health practitioners to make staff at all levels understand that patients/clients/customers must be served with a nonjudgmental attitude and respect. The word tolerance is often used when discussing attitudes toward other cultures, but the goal is to appreciate and value differences, not just to tolerate them. At the conclusion of the Assumption Exercise, participants should be asked the following questions, which they can ponder within the group and on their own:

- When was the first time you remember other people making you feel different?
- What were the circumstances of the situation?
- How did you feel as a consequence of this?
- How did you act on or deal with those feelings?

In a broader context, this preliminary phase of assessment enables participants of healthcare and public health organizations to determine a key aspect of their perspectives regarding difference and how it relates to cultural competence and to identify areas that need to be strengthened to ensure optimal outcomes in communicating and providing services.

CONCLUSIONS

Essentially, health service administrators and public health practitioners have a responsibility to delve into their organizations and explore the notion of the Cultural Competence Continuum. Organizations should ask themselves where they are in terms of the continuum and whether it is necessary to strive higher. Healthcare organizations and public health entities owe it to themselves and the people they serve to ensure that valuing and appreciating various cultures is a key goal. Mere tolerance should not be the goal. In addition, every level within healthcare and public health organizations should understand that the more information provided regarding various cultures, the better, and understanding of the Cultural Competence Continuum, the Cultural Competence Framework, and parameters that differentiate cultures is a good starting point. The Assumption Exercise, as a preliminary assessment process to foster dialogue, can initiate necessary analysis regarding the importance of cultural competence.

CHAPTER SUMMARY

The Cultural Competence Continuum consists of six levels; these are cultural destructiveness, cultural incapacity, cultural blindness, cultural precompetence, cultural competence, and cultural proficiency. The Cultural Competence Continuum is beneficial in enabling healthcare organizations and public health entities to determine their level of cultural competence and what steps should be considered to achieve cultural proficiency, which is the ultimate goal. Additionally, the Cultural Competence Framework consists of five components; these are cultural awareness, cultural knowledge, cultural skill, cultural encounters, and cultural desires. These constructs are important to begin to change the paradigm for healthcare organizations and public health entities from that of not understanding the importance of cultural competence to the point of embracing it based on practicality in terms of knowledge and skills. Furthermore, parameters that differentiate cultures offer insight into distinct differences that one can learn and understand, leading to valuing and appreciating other cultures and quelling concerns that may be based on lack of knowledge. Some of the key parameters are views of time and space and gender roles in different cultures. This knowledge and understanding will enable better provision of services and respect for the dynamics of differences. Ultimately, preliminary qualitative assessment must take place to explore key assumptions that individuals may have regarding differences among people based on appearances, languages, cultures, and stereotypes. One recommended approach is the Assumption Exercise, which is a process of looking at carefully selected images of individuals and, without thinking, immediately reacting in a brief written format to the images and then determining what assumptions have been made. Sometimes, assumptions are made that are inaccurate based on lack of information and understanding, and the best way to explore this is through candid dialogue and discussion with the help of an expert facilitator.

CHAPTER PROBLEMS

1. The president of a healthcare facility announces that all personnel at the hospital are to treat every person the same and that there are no inherent differences between one group of people and another. He indicates that although there has been a request for a cultural competence and diversity committee, he does not see the need for it, and all matters involving cultural and diversity concerns are to be handled by Human Resources. Based on this statement, at what level of the Cultural Competence Continuum would this organization be placed?

2. An outbreak of cholera is found in a remote area of a Native American community. Four White American public health workers are asked to visit the area for a series of meetings to discuss the issues with the community leaders. The third meeting is set for 5:00 PM. The community leaders show up at 5:30 PM. The public health workers are outraged because they have waited for what they deem to be an inordinate amount of time and this is not the first time that meetings have started late in this community with the public health workers. The community leaders are unapologetic about the time delay and are ready for discussion when they arrive. What should be explored in terms of the times of future meetings and perceptions of time delays?

3. During an Assumption Exercise at a cultural competence session with healthcare administrators at an American College of Healthcare Executives workshop, a picture is shown of an Asian American woman with a camera. Audience members are asked to anonymously write down their immediate impression in responding to the question, "Who is she?" In reviewing the responses, the group facilitator indicates that

the woman in the photograph has been labeled, in written anonymous responses by the audience, as a tourist, Korean, a Chinese tourist, and similar descriptions. The group is advised by the facilitator that the woman is actually a Japanese American Scientist working on a research project for the National Institutes of Health. What type of discussion should ensue about the assumptions made about the woman?

4. Think of a time in your life when you were made to feel different by others? How did you feel? What was your reaction? What did you want those who made you feel different to know about you?

5. A public health practitioner is in a largely Cuban community in Miami, Florida, gathering data from women regarding encouraging their spouses to use condoms to avoid unprotected sex. The women are advised to give their husbands information and encourage them to follow-up with their physicians for sexually transmitted disease testing. The women are very resistant and express discomfort in discussing these matters with their spouses. What information might be helpful to the public health workers in terms of their approach to this matter?

6. There are six levels of the Cultural Competence Continuum. Review each and discuss how a health service administrator might begin to ensure that his or her organization reaches the most positive end of the continuum. What is the ultimate goal, in terms of the continuum, and why?

REFERENCES

Campinha-Bacote, J. (1999). A model and instrument for addressing cultural competence in health care. *Journal of Nursing Education, 38,* 204–207.

Cross, T., Bazron, B., Dennis, K., & Isaacs, M. (1989). *Towards a culturally competent system of care* (Vol. 1). Washington, DC: Child and Adolescent Service System Program Technical Assistance Center, Center for Child and Mental Health Policy, Georgetown University Child Development Center.

Masson, V. (2005). Here to be seen: Ten practical lessons in cultural consciousness in primary health care. *Journal of Cultural Diversity, 12*(3), 94–98.

SUGGESTED READINGS

Lecca, P. (1998). *Cultural competency in health, social and human services: Directions for the 21st century.* Florence, KY: Routledge.

Orlandi, M. (1998). *Cultural competence for evaluators: A guide for drug abuse and other drug abuse prevention practitioners.* Washington, DC: US Department of Health and Human Services.

Srivastava, R. (2006). *The health care professional's guide to cultural competence.* New York: Elsevier Health Sciences.

Chapter 6

Cultural Competence and the Role of the Board of Directors, Health Service Administrators, Providers, and Staff

LEARNING OBJECTIVES

After reading this chapter, you should be able to:

- Explain the roles of the board of directors, health service administrators, providers, and staff regarding cultural competence.
- Discuss how to set standards, create policies, develop action plans, and allocate resources to support program initiatives regarding cultural competence.
- Describe processes including assessment, implementation, education/ training, and meeting legislative, regulatory, and accreditation mandates.
- Understand cultural competency as a priority for healthcare and public health organizations and as a way to maintain a competitive business advantage.

KEY TERMS

Council on Education for Public Health (CEPH)	Mission

INTRODUCTION

The purpose of this chapter is to focus on the roles of the board of directors, health service administrators, providers, and staff regarding cultural competence, which include setting standards and policies, development of action plans, allocation and reallocation of resources to support program initiatives, assessment, implementation, education/training, and meeting legislative, regulatory, and accreditation mandates. Emphasis is placed on the need for the process of cultural competence to begin at the top level of an organization, with a commitment from the board of directors and executives to ensure workforce diversity and the development of relevant policies specific to cultural competence initiatives. A case study will be discussed that involves a cultural competence program implemented at the Jessie Trice Community Health Center (JTCHC), Inc., an organization located in Miami, Florida. Using this case study, possible outcomes of such initiatives will be explored, including gaining a competitive edge in the marketplace; increasing market share and potential profitability; decreasing the likelihood of liability/malpractice claims; ensuring effective responses to current and projected demographic changes in the United States; eliminating long-standing disparities in the health status of people of diverse racial, ethnic, and cultural backgrounds; and ultimately improving the quality of services and health outcomes. The chapter will conclude with an overview of why cultural competence must be a priority for healthcare and public health organizations and how its effectiveness can be enriched while maintaining a competitive business advantage.

THE BOARD OF DIRECTORS

Culturally, and from a diversity standpoint, the board of directors of a healthcare organization should ideally be a representative microcosm of the community the organization serves. The board must consider the diversity of the community its organization serves and strive to become culturally competent for its population. One step in this direction is appointing of members from diverse backgrounds and reassessing the makeup of the board over time as community demographics change.

THE CHIEF EXECUTIVE OFFICER

The board of directors should strive to choose a chief executive officer (CEO) who best reflects the board's directives as they relate to successful administration in achieving its partnership with the community. The board should also consciously make an effort to hire a CEO who embraces the diverse nature of the community. When such a leader is hired, the bond between the institution and community is strengthened. The CEO, as the face of the institution, will be involved in community outreach and sets the tone to be followed by all subordinates in the hierarchical order of the organization (administrators, providers, managers, supervisors, and staff). The mission and vision statements of the organization should state the organization's dedication and commitment to serving the needs of a diverse population, and it is the CEO who must lead the organization toward that goal.

MISSION

The **mission** of an organization is generally formulated into a brief statement that indicates why the organization exists and states the purpose of the organization. Once the mission is declared, it is incumbent upon all levels of management to embrace the goal of achieving cultural competence as part of the strategic plan. It is at the administrative level that policy is then created, interpreted, and implemented in an effort to meet the organization's mission (Cross, Bazron, Dennis, & Isaacs, 1989). Human resources and staff education departments should lead the development of criteria concerning cultural competence for the hiring and educating of the institution's employees at all levels. An organization can begin with a self-assessment and a review of its patient/client/customer demographics to aid in planning its direction (Cross et al., 1989). By focusing on patient/client/customer demographics, cultural competence training can be used to the best advantage of the institution and should be marketed to the community at some level when the time is appropriate. Processes within the organization should be reviewed and implemented along culturally competent lines. Existing services should be adapted to fit the needs of those who are served, based on identity, degree of assimilation, and subcultural grouping (Cross et al., 1989).

STAFF

Within healthcare and public health institutions, it is not only processes that must be adapted to embrace cultural competency, but also people, who become ambassadors of the processes in their roles as frontline staff. These individuals must also adapt to becoming culturally competent. By using the process of assessment, organizations can rate levels of cultural competence and then educate staff based on their status and the needs of the community. An assessment enables an organization to determine what it is doing well in terms of cultural competence, identifies any gaps, and allows for the creation of an agenda for improving its services based on gathered data. There must be a commitment from leadership to carefully review the organization's assessment and implement training to improve identified weakness. Individuals from the community are excellent resources and can be used as training "experts" in some instances (Cross et al., 1989).

Additionally, it cannot be expected that every individual within an organization will be culturally competent, based on their race or ethnicity, in the cultural group they appear to represent because there are so many regional differences within groups. For example, it cannot be assumed that just because a person is African American, he or she is culturally competent regarding African American culture; he or she may not have in-depth insight into the African American culture or may be from a particular region that maintains a distinct culture. Specifically, an African American from the south may have a very different cultural perspective from an African American who lives in the north. Staff should acknowledge that regardless of their culture, clients from various cultures will often have very different customs from their own, and when staff cannot be of assistance to a particular group, they should know where to seek help. Organizations should set up a cultural resource center that can be accessed by staff members, practitioners, or patients to address their needs. Culturally competent programs within health service and public health organizations should be viewed as "living, breathing entities" in that they must change over time as the demographics of the patients/clients/customers change.

ACCREDITATION

For a healthcare or public health organization to function effectively in terms of cultural competence, standards, policies, and procedures must be established that represent a clear understanding of specific needs to ensure efficacious care for those being served. This includes ensuring respect for patients/clients/customers, recognizing the need for a diverse and trained staff, understanding the demographics of those being served, and establishing leadership that is committed to cultural competence. Such commitment includes translation of all pertinent materials, language interpretation, visual affirmation, and so on. However, to ensure that all of these measures are present, accrediting bodies have begun requiring that healthcare facilities meet certain standards specific to cultural competence. For example, The Joint Commission now requires adherence to standards specific to culture.

Cultural competence reflects the belief that each patient/client/customer is an individual with specific needs that are often culturally based. To that end, the Joint Commission standards that are relevant to culture are designed to ensure that these needs are met, both on a broad basis and individually. The Joint Commission's accreditation process determines compliance with certain standards based on a number of processes including observation by Joint Commission surveyors, documentation, and verbal communication with staff to determine their understanding of the specific requirements of given standards (The Joint Commission, 1998). As of August of 2008, The Joint Commission, with funding received from the Commonwealth Fund, began the process of developing standards that are specific to cultural competence rather than implied. Previously, cultural standards were in place but were somewhat vague and nonspecific. For example, from the standards published in the Assessment of Patients, the following standard, Standard PF. 1.7, has the implication of addressing cultural competence: "Patients are informed about access to additional resources in the community" (The Joint Commission, 1998). This standard indirectly relates to cultural competence in that it implies that there are resources that an individual may need that go beyond what the healthcare organization may have to offer. This may include cultural resources or others.

Another example of an implied culturally relevant Joint Commission standard is Standard RI.1.3 published in Patient Rights: "The hospital demonstrates respect for the following patient needs (RI.1.2.1) confidentiality, (RI.1.3.2) privacy, (RI 1.3.5) pastoral counseling and (RI 1.3.6) communication" (The Joint Commission, 1998). This standard is an example of implied relevance to cultural competence because it may be assumed that cultures handle matters of privacy, confidentiality, and so on differently. Consequently, the standard ensures that healthcare organizations consider these matters on a broad and individual basis, which perhaps will include the notion of culture in the process.

The new standards currently in the process of development by The Joint Commission will be specifically related to culture and language and will ensure that these matters will be directly assessed. The new standards will be entitled the *Culturally Competent Patient-Centered Care Standards* and will extend the research that was conducted by the Joint Commission (2007) entitled *Hospitals, Language and Culture: A Snapshot of the Nation*. The projected time frame for the development of the new standards is from August 2008 through January 2010. Some of the issues that the project will explore include how to incorporate diversity, culture, language, and health literacy into current Joint Commission standards. Participation in this project includes an expert advisory panel from a number of disciplines who represent a broad range of stakeholders.

COUNCIL ON EDUCATION FOR PUBLIC HEALTH

Another accrediting body relevant to the field of health, specifically public health, is the **Council on Education for Public Health (CEPH)**, which provides accreditation for institutions that prepare graduates for public health practice. The primary purpose of CEPH accreditation is to ensure that excellence in public health education relates directly to proficiency in practice. Consequently, CEPH has developed specific criteria that must be met in order for a program or school to receive accreditation. However, do criteria exist within this accreditation framework that are relevant to cultural competence? There are certain characteristics that public health programs and schools have to demonstrate, including, but are not limited to, being part of an institution of higher education accredited by a regional accrediting body recognized by the US Department of Education; rights specific to faculty, instruction, research, and service; and a general embracement of public health, governance, financial, and learning resources. However, there are no characteristics, at this time, that are specific to cultural competence. The areas of knowledge the criteria focus on are biostatistics, epidemiology, environmental health sciences, health services administration, and social and behavioral sciences. To fully comprehend these knowledge areas and for public health schools and programs to function optimally, cultural competence should be outlined in unique and specific criteria given the demographic changes in the Unites States and the diversity public health practitioners will be exposed to in the United States and globally.

CEPH does include the requirement of faculty and staff diversity, indicating the necessity of requiring the recruitment, retention, and promotion of staff based on age, gender, race, disability, sexual orientation, religion, and national origin. However, because diversity and cultural competence are different concepts, ensuring diversity does not ensure cultural competence. The necessary skill sets need to be established for both faculty and students, even if they are from diverse demographic groups. Public health practitioners and administrators, per a Robert Wood Johnson Foundation study, have recognized the importance of diversity and cultural competence skills but indicate that a major barrier to the latter is limited time for training (Boedigheimer & Gebbie, 2001). Therefore, including such training in the curriculum of public health students may eliminate this hurdle. By including cultural competence as a criterion, perhaps CEPH can ensure that this happens.

Another association that has specific relevance to healthcare administrators is the American College of Healthcare Executives (ACHE). Although it is not an accrediting body, health service administrators look to the ACHE for guidance in terms of literature, information, and general insight, and thus, it is a substantial resource. At present, ACHE appears to focus primarily, although not exclusively, on diversity rather than cultural competence in terms of its literature. Per a review of the ACHE Web site, it appears that the main area of interest regarding diversity is the promotion of minorities in healthcare management. However, ACHE has offered several workshops at its annual conference in Chicago on the topic of cultural competence and its relevance to healthcare administrators, including several by the author of this text. The ACHE does seem to recognize the business case for cultural competence among healthcare administrators, and Brach and Fraser (2002) have identified at least four financial incentives to implement cultural competence initiatives. These four incentives are increasing appeal to consumers, competing for private purchaser business, responding to private purchaser demands, and improving cost and effectiveness (Brach & Fraser). Along with the acknowledgement of the incentives, Brach and Fraser also voice concerns about costs pertaining to culturally competence initiatives. Nevertheless, as a result of demographic changes, there is a need for services based on familiarity with other cultures, and the relevance to the business of health care must be an ongoing concern.

SETTING STANDARDS, CREATING POLICIES, AND RESOURCE ALLOCATION: A CASE STUDY

The Jessie Trice Community Health Center, Inc., (JTCHC), formerly the Economic Opportunity Family Health Center, Inc. (EOFHC), is a community health center and major provider of quality healthcare services in Miami, Florida, that serves a multicultural and multilingual population comprised of African American, Haitian, Caribbean, Latin and Central American, and Caucasian people (Table 6-1). JTCHC has consistently maintained Joint Commission accreditation. As one of the nation's oldest, most comprehensive, and largest community health centers, the organization faces challenges specifically related to the delivery of healthcare, behavioral health, and social services. It is essentially a comprehensive entity that meets the primary care, public health, and health education needs of the community it serves.

Table 6-1 Economic Opportunity Family Health Center Patient Demographics in 2001[a]

Race/Ethnicity	Percentage of Patients
Haitian	10%
Hispanic	20%
Caribbean	5%
African American	60%
Caucasian	5%

[a] The Economic Opportunity Family Health Center is now known as the Jessie Trice Community Health Center.

Source: Economic Opportunity Family Health Center (EOFHC). (2001). *Annual report, 2001.* Miami, FL.

In an effort to establish cultural competence at all levels of JTCHC, the CEO made a decision, with the support of the board of directors, to take on an ambitious cultural competence initiative (Munroe & Rose, 2003). The notion to incorporate cultural competence into its service delivery framework was a bold move fiscally and as a change initiative. The goal was to ensure that the board of directors and every employee at the organization (including health service administrators and providers) would acquire the necessary knowledge concerning cultural competence and to put it into practice at every level of the organization.

Planning and Action

Deliberate and detailed cultural competence planning was undertaken by the JTCHC (then the EOFHC) in 2003. It was a venture into unchartered territory because the approach was aggressive, comprehensive, and tailored to the needs of the staff and community and cultural competence was not yet established in many community health centers throughout the nation. The Office of Minority Health of the Department of Health and Human Services released the final national standards on Culturally and Linguistically Appropriate Services (CLAS) for healthcare organizations on December 22, 2000. The final CLAS standards, to be discussed in detail in Chapter 9, were announced in the *Federal Register* and were the first of their kind in the US healthcare system. Some of the standards are mandates, whereas others are guidelines and recommendations.

Subsequent to review of these standards, through an overview provided by a consultant (the author of this text) to initiate and implement the process, the CEO made frequent public statements about the organization's plans to implement a cultural competence program with the goal of meeting the diverse needs of the patient/client/customer population based on their cultural backgrounds to be determined by the collection of demographic data. This was an important step because it provided a clear and resounding message to staff at every level of the organization that initiation and support for this effort began at the top of the organization; in essence, the CEO was selling cultural competence to the organization. The CEO made it clear that this was a new vision for the organization and that cultural competence would be incorporated into its mission statement, polices, practices, and attitudes.

Once the vision of cultural competence was sold to the organization by the CEO, the next step was implementation, which took place in phases. The first phase consisted of the following steps:

- A comprehensive cultural competence assessment of the board of directors, executives (including the CEO), providers, and all levels of staff.

- Development and delivery of cultural competence training sessions/ workshops for the board of directors, executives, providers, and all levels of staff.

The second phase consisted of a substantial implementation process that included the following steps:

- Provision of creative and innovative mechanisms for the dissemination of ongoing information relevant to cultural competence (e.g., a cultural competence newsletter entitled *The Cultural Voice*) and plans to include information on the organization's Web site.
- Quantitative and qualitative data collection and analysis.
- Revision of the mission statement of the organization to include culturally and linguistically appropriate language.
- Development of a cultural competence policy.
- Translation of patient education material, marketing materials, and signage into Spanish and Creole.
- Inclusion of cultural competence training in the new employee orientation and annual employee training.
- Acquisition and display of culturally relevant artwork, at all sites, to ensure visual affirmation of clients served.
- Use of a language line and a language bank to ensure interpretation availability to prevent language barriers in the provision of services.

Assessment, Education, and Training

Although the cultural competence assessment process will be discussed in detail in Chapter 7, it is important to discuss some highlights of it here in relation to the JTCHC case study. At JTCHC, three distinct surveys were developed by selecting questions from existing cultural competence tools and developing new questions that were specifically relevant to the organization (see Appendices I, II, and III). A survey was developed for the executive team and management (also used for the board of directors), staff at all levels, and providers. Reliability and validity of the tools were established through the hiring of a statistician (consultant). Response categories were based on a Likert-type format of strongly agree, agree, strongly disagree, disagree, and N/A (not applicable), and the surveys focused on the assessment of attitudes. Numerical scores were assigned for each response category, and data were analyzed based on the following categories: concern for others, self-awareness, patient contact, cultural sensitivity, workshops/training, knowledge, and communication and language.

Analysis of data yielded specific strengths and weaknesses among the various groups assessed regarding their culturally competent attitudes; a need for training/workshops was identified in the areas of concern for others, self-awareness, cultural sensitivity, knowledge, and communication and language (linguistic competency). Employees indicated that they found it difficult to or did not want to communicate with patients/clients/customers who could not speak English, which was deemed a significant weakness.

Assessment is extremely important because it provides insight into culturally relevant development needs of staff, as was the case at JTCHC. Workshops and training were developed and offered to address the cultural competence needs of JTCHC staff. Board members, executives, staff at all levels, and providers participated in training that was specifically tailored to meet their needs. Sessions such as "Elements of a Culturally Proficient System of Care," "Issues of Relevance to Cultural/Ethnic Groups in South Florida," "Eliminating Stereotypes," and "Universal Principles for Communicating with Patients/Clients" were some of the training sessions and workshops offered. Individuals were provided with Certificates of Achievement to reward their successful completion of training, which were placed in their personnel file, recognizing their acquisition of new knowledge regarding cultural competence.

INITIATIVES

Approaches to maintaining excitement around cultural competence must be established. An idea that surfaced at JTCHC was the development of a newsletter entitled *The Cultural Voice*. The purpose of the newsletter was to provide ongoing information and updates on issues relevant to cultural competence from a local and national vantage point, commentary from the CEO, and articles written by the staff and community. The newsletter also served to announce cultural events at JTCHC and in the community, culturally relevant national and federal policies, accreditation requirements, resource lists, and cultural recipes and historical notes, which are fun and culturally informative components that allow staff and community members to share important aspects of their cultural heritage. Board members, employees, patients/clients/customers, and community members are encouraged to submit entries to the newsletter as an empowering mechanism so their voices can be heard regarding cultural matters of importance to them. Thus, a reciprocal relationship of providing and receiving cultural information was established.

CONCLUSIONS

Although JTCHC is merely one example of a healthcare organization that provides a comprehensive approach to cultural competence for a healthcare organization, it serves as a benchmark for addressing and responding to the various challenges faced by healthcare organizations regarding cultural competence. The goal for healthcare organizations, as a starting point, is to attempt to meet the CLAS standards, to address specific requirements of accreditation entities that are beginning to understand the need for cultural competence standards and criteria, and to respond to ongoing demographic changes that reflect the tremendous diversity of American society. Most importantly, cultural competence programs should be comprehensive, cutting edge, and clearly documented so that they are replicable by other organizations that are willing to proceed in this direction. Because cultural competence initiatives are relatively new for healthcare and public health organizations, outcome data are limited. Nevertheless, as these organizations begin to experience successes, they should be documented and shared so that others can explore the information and use the data as benchmarks to assess their own achievements.

CHAPTER SUMMARY

Without a doubt, healthcare organizations have an ethical obligation to provide culturally congruent care to all individuals who enter their facilities and to those who are recipients of public health efforts, no matter the venue. To ensure success, the board of directors, CEO, staff, providers, and public health practitioners at every level must be involved. Open minds and creativity are necessary because limited resources often present a barrier to implementation of cultural competence efforts. However, if cultural competence is incorporated into the very fabric of healthcare organizations and public health entities, including standards, policies, action plans, and allocation of resources, and mechanisms are put in place to reward and document successes and ensure that regulatory, legislative, and accreditation requirements are met regarding cultural competence, then surely the provision of services will be enhanced while, at the same time, organizations will obtain a competitive business advantage.

CHAPTER PROBLEMS

1. A healthcare organization has decided to incorporate a cultural competence initiative into the fabric of the organization. You have been hired as a consultant to begin this process. What initial steps would you recommend?

2. In an effort to be creative and to keep information regarding cultural competence at the forefront of the organization's ongoing activities, a healthcare organization has implemented the production and distribution of a newsletter that specifically addresses cultural issues relevant to the facility. What other ideas might be useful to continue to stimulate interest in cultural competence? Suggest at least three innovative and creative ideas.

3. Although a CEO is convinced that cultural competence will be a great addition to her hospital's initiatives, she realizes that such an endeavor will be costly, and given current financial shortfalls, there is a concern about whether the board of directors will share her view. What approach might she take to convince the board that this will be a worthwhile endeavor?

4. A public health effort in a small migrant community of Mexican people that includes brochures and posters that are to be distributed is in the developmental stages. Public health workers will develop and distribute the materials. In terms of cultural competence, what factors should be taken into consideration regarding this effort?

5. A CEPH accreditation team is planning to visit a public health program that is seeking to advance its status from a program to a school. In terms of cultural competence and diversity, what should be taken into consideration in order to meet CEPH criteria?

REFERENCES

Boedigheimer, S. F., & Gebbie, K. M. (2001). Currently employed public health administrators: Are they prepared? *Journal of Public Health Management and Practice,* *7*(1), 30–36.

Brach, C., & Fraser, I. (2002). Reducing disparities through culturally competent health care: An analysis of the business case. *Quality Management in Health Care,* *10*(4), 15–28.

Cross, T., Bazron, B., Dennis, K., & Isaacs, M. (1989). *Towards a culturally competent system of care* (Vol. 1, pp. 28–31). Washington, DC: Child and Adolescent Service System Program Technical Assistance Center, Center for Child and Mental Health Policy, Georgetown University Child Development Center.

Munroe, A., & Rose, P. (2003). A benchmark for the future: The national cultural proficiency model of the economic opportunity family health center. *Vital Signs,* *13*(2), 12–13.

The Joint Commission. (1998). *Hospital accreditation standards.* Oakbrook Terrace, IL: Author.

The Joint Commission. (2007). *Hospitals, language and culture: A snapshot of the nation.* Retrieved November 18, 2009, from http://www.jointcommission.org/NR/rdonlyres/E64E5E89-5734-4D1D-BB4D-C4ACD4BF8BD3/0/hlc_paper.pdf.

SUGGESTED READINGS

Rundle, A., Carvalho, M., & Robinson, M. (Eds.). (2002). *Cultural competence in healthcare: A practical guide*. Indianapolis, IN: Jossey-Bass.

Swayne, L., Duncan, J., & Ginter, P. (2007). *Strategic management of healthcare organizations* (5th ed.). Malden, MA: Blackwell Publishing.

The Joint Commission. (2005). *Providing culturally and linguistically competent health care*. Oakbrook Terrace, IL: Author.

Tseng, W., & Strelzer, J. (2008). *Cultural competence in healthcare*. New York: Springer.

Chapter 7

Cultural Competency and Assessment

LEARNING OBJECTIVES

After reading this chapter, you should be able to:

- Understand assessment in terms of health care.
- Explain the relevance of measuring attitudes of health service administrators, board members, providers, and staff and public health practitioners of organizations serving diverse populations.
- Discuss the importance of establishing reliability and validity of cultural competency assessment tools.
- Determine the usefulness of data in training and other plans for organizations.

┌─ **KEY TERMS** ─────────────────────────

Alternative form reliability	Internal consistency
Construct validity	Lack of clarity
Content validity	Lack of complexity
Convergent validity	Reliability
Criterion validity	Test-retest reliability
Divergent validity	Validity
Face validity	

INTRODUCTION

This chapter will focus on assessment and cultural competence in an effort to explain the relevance of measuring attitudes of health service administrators, board members, providers, staff, and public health practitioners of organizations serving diverse populations. In general, assessment determines the cultural competence preparedness of individuals who work in health service/public health organizations. The use of an attitudinal assessment tool, with established reliability and validity, is one approach to determine the level of cultural competence preparedness. An overview of the importance of reliability and validity of cultural competence assessment tools is provided, and the significance of reassessment on a consistent basis and why survey data are useful in implementation of training and other plans for health service and public health organizations are discussed.

ATTITUDES

Healthcare organizations and public health entities that serve diverse populations must be cognizant of their attitudes within the context of serving various cultures. This awareness must take place at every level of organizations, including board members, administrators, providers, staff, and public health practitioners. An approach to measuring such attitudes is the use of carefully designed, reliable, and valid instruments or surveys specifically focused on cultural competence and its various constructs. Negative attitudes, from a cultural vantage point, may lead to lack of efficacy in terms of care, poor communication, loss of customers, and a host of other problems. These problems can be avoided if attitudinal deficits are properly assessed and training to change these negative attitudes is enacted. The first step in assessment is to use tools that are specifically designed for various groups, including board members, administrators, providers, and staff. A survey will yield useful results that healthcare and public health organizations can use to strengthen any attitudinal weaknesses regarding cultural competence in order to provide better services to all people.

ASSESSMENT

Surveys are an inherently social activity and are generally used to ask respondents about their behaviors, attitudes, and beliefs; thus, they are conducive to the cultural competence assessment process. Part of the assessment process for investigators is to evaluate how well a survey instrument measures what it is intended to measure. The **reliability** of a survey refers to the stability and equivalence of measures of the same concept over time or across methods of gathering data. Reliability is commonly assessed using a number of methods, including test–retest reliability, alternative form reliability, and internal consistency. Additionally, in terms of efficacy, validity, lack of complexity, and lack of clarity of the instrument are important. **Validity** refers to the consistency of the results of the measure, **lack of complexity** refers to how easy the instrument is to administer, and **lack of clarity** refers to whether or not the survey questions are vague or ambiguous.

Test–Retest Reliability

Test–retest reliability is conducted to determine whether an instrument will measure what it is purported to measure, from time 1 to time 2. The instrument is given to the same group of respondents once and then repeated a second time within a reasonable interim of time (no more than 2 weeks). Statistical measures—correlation coefficients—are used to determine whether, from time 1 to time 2, the results are stable and the results correlate. If the coefficient is closer to $+1.0$, then the test responses are said to be stable (Aday, 1996). If the coefficient is below 0.70, then the test-retest reliability coefficient is generally considered too low (Litwin, 1995; Alwin, 1989).

Alternative Form Reliability

Alternative form reliability is the utilization of differently worded items to measure the same attribute. Thus, the original survey's questions and responses are reworded to produce a second instrument that is similar but not identical to the first. In this process, correlation coefficients are also calculated in an effort to acquire a measure indicative of the two instruments. If the coefficients are high, the instrument is said to have good alternative form reliability. A coefficient of 0.70 or greater indicates high reliability.

Internal Consistency Reliability

Another measure of reliability is **internal consistency**, which is a determination of the performance levels of various aspects of the same concept. Instruments are designed to measure certain constructs that are comprised of various questions or items. Internal consistency examines the questions or items pertaining to a given construct/concept to determine whether the results are consistent using measures such as interitem correlation, average item total correlation, split-half reliability, and Cronbach's alpha (Aday, 1996). Although these statistical concepts are beyond the scope of this text, these measures suffice in the analysis process to determine internal consistency reliability.

Validity

There are four types of validity measures: face, content, criterion, and construct. **Face validity** entails a review of the items by individuals who are not trained in the survey development process. The process involves showing the survey to individuals and asking them what they think of it. It is clearly the least scientific approach to establishing validity (Litwin, 1995). Theoretically, there is no limit to the number of questions that could be asked about attitudes in terms of cultural competence. However, certain concepts should be explored by the questions; thus, the questions should be representative of the concepts they are intended to reflect because only a sampling of questions can be included in the instrument. Therefore, **content validity** refers to the sampling adequacy of the items used to measure the subject matter. Furthermore, another measure, **criterion validity**, provides quantitative evidence of the accuracy of a survey instrument (Litwin, 1995).

There are two types of content validity: predictive and construct. As implied by the term, predictive validity uses the survey results as a predictor based on the assumption that if the prediction result is accurate, the instrument is presumed valid (Weisberg & Restuccia, 1989). This process requires the use of a "gold standard" for assessing the same variable (Litwin, 1995; Aday, 1996). The Pearson correlation coefficient, another statistical measure, is used to indicate the strength of performance of both predictive and concurrent validity measures. Criterion-related strategy is concerned with examining the systematic relationship (usually in the form of a correlation coefficient) between scores on a given scale and other scores it should predict.

Construct validity asks the following question about an instrument: Does the instrument measure the theoretical framework that it is designed to measure? Implied in this inquiry is that there are theories and/ or hypotheses about the relationship of a particular variable to other variables measured in the study. Two forms of construct validity are convergent and divergent validity (Weisberg & Restuccia, 1989). Essentially, measures of the same concept should receive similar answers (convergent validity), whereas measures of different concepts should receive different answers (discriminant or divergent validity). **Convergent validity** implies that several different methods for obtaining the same information about a given concept produce similar results. **Divergent validity**

is assessed by comparing a respondent's answer to a question measuring one concept to the respondent's answer to a question intended to measure a different concept; if divergent validity is present, the answers will be different.

A CULTURAL COMPETENCE ASSESSMENT TOOL

In an effort to assess cultural competence attitudes, a cultural competence tool was developed by the author of this text. Three distinct surveys were developed based on questions that are particularly relevant to healthcare organizations. (See Appendices I to III for the three surveys.) The surveys were designed to assess boards of directors, executive teams, and managers; providers; and staff. The response categories are based on a Likert-type format of strongly agree, agree, strongly disagree, disagree, and N/A (not applicable), enabling numerical score assignment for each of the following seven content response categories: (1) concern for others, (2) self-awareness, (3) patient/client/customer contact, (4) cultural sensitivity, (5) workshops/training, (6) knowledge, and (7) communication and language.

In an effort to establish reliability and validity, a study was conducted involving four stages. The first stage was to review and evaluate the survey tool. The next stage was survey data collection, followed by data entry. The last stage was statistical analysis. Several methods, as described earlier, were used to measure reliability and validity. Test–retest, alternative form, and Cronbach's alpha estimate (internal consistency) were used to test reliability. Content-related strategy and construct-related strategy were used to test validity. All survey tools passed the rigorous statistical tests for reliability and validity. Based on parallel form, the average estimates for reliability were 0.81 for the executive survey (0.72 for the board of directors), 0.71 for the provider survey, and 0.77 for the staff survey. Additionally, the Cronbach's alpha estimates were all within the acceptable range of > 0.7 for all survey instruments. Finally, all surveys demonstrated good content, construct, and item-discriminant validity.

IMPORTANCE OF RELIABLE AND VALID ASSESSMENT TOOLS

Surveys are important tools to gather data, but without established reliability and validity, survey results have little or no meaning. Healthcare and public health organizations are often unaware of or have very little insight into the attitudes and perspectives of their members, at every level, in terms of cultural competence. Gaining insight, through the use of a survey tool, is useful to determine what areas of weakness may benefit from targeted training efforts to improve staff attitudes regarding important cultural competence constructs. Tailoring the surveys to specifically address the hierarchical level of the organization ensures that queries are specific to the correct intended respondents. Often, by merely responding to items on an attitudinal survey, respondents gain insight regarding cultural competence as they explore questions that they may not have considered previously. A number of factors may influence attitudes over time, such as education, socioeconomic status, and personality traits, so it is important to reassess attitudes on an ongoing and consistent basis to ensure that negative attitudes are addressed through training and workshops that are specifically geared to address areas of concern.

CONCLUSIONS

It is imperative that survey tools that are designed to measure attitudes toward cultural competence and its relevant constructs have established reliability and validity. There are many measures to establish reliability and validity, which is essential to ensure that the survey data are relevant and useful. Consequently, upon review of the survey data, training sessions can be developed to address areas of attitudinal weakness, in terms of cultural competence, for all levels of healthcare and public health organizations.

CHAPTER SUMMARY

In the fields of public health and health services administration, cultural competence assessment is important to acquire data and determine areas of weakness to ensure that training is provided to strengthen identified areas of concern. Measuring attitudes is a good approach because it provides a sense of individuals views about the provision of services to patients/clients/customers who are from varying cultural backgrounds. When conducting such attitudinal research, every level of the organization should be assessed, including the board of directors, executives, providers, staff, and public health practitioners, because all individuals in an organization impact health services provision. Any assessment tool used must have established reliability and validity to ensure the efficacy of the data collected. There are a number of approaches for establishing reliability and validity. Once methods for doing so are determined, the process should be conducted methodically and accurately to ensure that findings from the data can be used to determine what type of cultural competence training is needed to improve organizational attitudes. Assessment should be conducted on a regular basis (perhaps annually) to ensure that positive attitudes regarding serving diverse populations remain intact with the provision of training as necessary, based on the data, if there are changes or concerns that arise.

CHAPTER PROBLEMS

1. A healthcare organization serves a diverse community in the inner city of Boston that consists of African American, Cape Verdean, and Hispanic members. The staff, of which the majority are White, are concerned because they know little about the cultures of the groups they are working with. What should be an important step for the organization when establishing a plan to provide the staff with cultural competence training?
2. A public health supervisor with interest in determining attitudes of staff at his organization decides to draft a 10-item questionnaire to determine perspectives regarding cultural competence. He drafts the questions, photocopies them, calls a meeting, and asks the staff to complete the survey during the meeting. He collects the surveys, reviews the questions, and decides that training is needed immediately and hires a consultant. Is this an effective cultural competence survey process?
3. What measures are used to determine reliability of a survey instrument?
4. List at least three validity measures for a survey instrument.
5. An administrator of a healthcare organization hires a consultant to develop a survey to measure attitudes of staff regarding cultural competence. The consultant agrees to develop the survey following appropriate measures to establish reliability and validity. The survey is to be administered to the board of directors, the executive team, providers, and staff. The consultant develops one form of the survey and explains to the administrator that it will be sufficient to use at all of the various levels. Is this the correct approach for this survey process?

References

Aday, L. U. (1996). *Designing and conducting health surveys: A comprehensive guide* (2nd ed.). San Francisco: Jossey-Bass.

Alwin, D. F. (1989). Problems in the estimation and interpretation of the reliability of survey data. *Quality and Quantity, 23,* 277–331.

Litwin, M. S. (1995). *How to measure survey reliability.* Thousand Oaks, CA: Sage Publications.

Weisberg, H. F., & Restuccia, J. D. (1989). *An introduction to survey research and data analysis* (2nd ed.). Glenview, IL: Scott, Foresman and Company.

SUGGESTED READINGS

Kuzma, J. (1998). *Basic statistics for the health sciences.* Mountain View, CA: McGraw-Hill.

Scott, M. G. (2002). Cultural competency: How is it measured? Does it make a difference? *Generations, 26*(3), 39–45.

Chapter 8

Cultural Competence Training

LEARNING OBJECTIVES

After reading this chapter, you should be able to:

- Understand the significance of cultural competence training.
- Discuss the key components of training.
- Describe how to develop/identify necessary training programs.
- Explain the need for cross-cultural education.
- Define key terms relevant to the process of training.

┌─ **KEY TERMS** ──────────────────────────────

Attitude-based approaches   People of color

Cultural sensitivity   Skill-building approaches

Knowledge-based approaches   Stereotypes

└──

INTRODUCTION

The primary goal of this chapter is to highlight the significance of training the staff and administrators of health service and public health practitioners to ensure appropriate skill sets in serving diverse populations. The key components of training will be discussed, as well as approaches for developing and identifying training programs to specifically address the needs of the organization. The need for cross-cultural education will be emphasized along with essential elements of training, including an overview of health disparities, key terms relevant to cultural competence, cultural definitions of health and illness, and the need to integrate cultural competence into organizations. The importance of evaluating training programs will also be discussed.

THE SIGNIFICANCE OF CULTURAL COMPETENCE TRAINING

Formal, professional cultural competence training and education are important because they can help healthcare professionals avoid discriminatory practices even when racial bias and cultural insensitivity are not intended (Brathwaite & Majumdar, 2006). Health service administrators and public health practitioners should keep cultural competence training at the forefront of their organizations, with an emphasis on determining approaches that will be most beneficial to their patients/clients/customers, in an effort to eliminate the possibility of discriminatory and culturally and linguistically insensitive and inappropriate practices. Given the importance of cultural competence to healthcare organizations, cultural competence training should be undertaken within the context of the directional strategies and strategic plans for organizations.

APPROACHES TO TRAINING

Three approaches are relevant to the provision of cultural competence training and education. They are knowledge-based, attitude-based, and skill-building approaches. **Knowledge-based approaches** include specific information of relevance to cultural competence, including definitions of culture, race, ethnicity, linguistic competence, and related concepts; details about health-seeking behaviors of various cultures; and so on. **Attitude-based approaches** involve improving awareness of specific elements of attitudes, values, and beliefs regarding various cultures and of perspectives about language and other culturally and linguistically relevant factors that may impact the provision of optimal services to patients/clients/customers. **Skill-building approaches** involve the provision of training to develop specific skill sets that will prepare individuals with knowledge of how to communicate effectively with individuals who do not speak English, how to identify an interpreter when needed, and how to ensure that individuals feel valued and appreciated in terms of their culture based on discussions with them about cultural nuances when they enter a healthcare or public health facility.

Decisions regarding the best training approaches for a given organization are imperative and should be made based on weaknesses identified in the assessment process, as discussed in Chapter 7. Once approaches have been determined, the goal should be to ensure the success of training. For example, as a skill-building approach, once practical cultural competence skills have been taught, immediate feedback should be provided based on ongoing implementation of the skills. A feedback and evaluative approach should be undertaken for all aspects of training based on monitoring by quality improvement departments that track progress over time, while identifying short-term and long-term successes or shortcomings resulting from the training programs. Customer service evaluations can be effective tools to determine the impact of training if they include questions regarding the quality of culturally competent services.

ELEMENTS NEEDED TO ENSURE SUCCESSFUL TRAINING PROGRAMS

For training of cultural competence in healthcare and public health organizations to be successful, there has to be "buy-in" for such training from the leadership of the organization. This, and all other related endeavors, should begin with the board of directors. Although the board does not have patient/client/customer contact and is not involved in the day-to-day operations of the organization, it is helpful to provide all members with cultural competence education, based on the approaches mentioned earlier, to ensure that they understand the definition and merits of cultural competence. Executives, including the chief executive officer (CEO) and his or her team, and all other members of the organization should also be trained. The emphasis of their training should be to increase awareness of racial and ethnic health disparities, to ensure that human resources skills are developed for cross-cultural assessment, to learn how to communicate and negotiate from a cultural vantage point, to understand the significance of allocating resources to support cultural competence program initiatives, and to impart insight regarding the importance of developing institutional benchmarks and rewarding successes in terms of cultural competence. Training at this level should also focus on current accreditation requirements regarding cultural competence, as well as any state and/or federal requirements. Because emphasis in healthcare and public health organizations is often placed on diversity rather than cultural competence, the difference between diversity and cultural competence should be established, with explanation provided as to why it is necessary to diversify the workforce in addition to implementing cultural competence efforts. The best approaches to ensure a culturally diverse workforce and the importance of enhancing the skill sets of staff by including cultural competence training should be considered.

THE NEED FOR CROSS-CULTURAL EDUCATION AND OTHER TRAINING ESSENTIALS

Often, the question arises as to why cross-cultural education and cultural competence training are needed. According to the Institute of Medicine, education and training are needed to begin the process of addressing health disparities. People of color often experience discrimination regarding the provision of health care (Smedley, Stith, & Nelson, 2003). Essentially, **people of color** are individuals who are classified as being part of minority groups, namely Blacks or African Americans, Native Americans, Alaska Natives, Asians and Pacific Islanders, and Hispanics or Latinos. As mentioned in Chapter 2, Latino and Hispanic are ethnic rather than racial groups. Thus, regarding the term people of color, the discussion is relevant to Hispanics and Latinos who are not White.

Bias, prejudice, and stereotyping may impact the care provided to people seeking health services. Cultural competence training can bring attention to these potential occurrences and eliminate them. Regarding linguistic competency, cultural competence training can help members of healthcare and public health organizations understand that in the United States, the number of people who are not proficient in English is growing rapidly. Linguistic isolation is a problem particularly among the Hispanic, Latino, and Asian and Pacific Islander populations. Many languages are spoken in the United States. According to the 2003 US Census, the languages spoken in the United States, other than English, include Spanish, Asian/Pacific Island languages, Indo-European languages, and languages classified as other. Individuals will often forego care when language obstacles are present. Therefore, training in universal approaches of communicating with individuals who are not proficient in English is a very helpful component of cultural competence training.

Additionally, cultural competence training can provide knowledge of key terms and aspects of cultural competence including, but not limited to, ethnicity, race, culture, religion, socioeconomic status, and gender. Cultural competence training should also provide information regarding behavioral norms based on culture and cultural factors. Training needs to be ongoing and updated often because culture is not stagnant; it constantly changes. Cultural training should include exercises that cause participants to think and participate in active learning. Formats should include lectures, role playing, use of audiovisual material pertaining to cultural competence, group dynamics, and discussion/dialogue. Participants should be encouraged to share their own cultures as part of the teaching–learning process.

THE IMPORTANCE OF PROVIDING KEY TERMS RELEVANT TO CULTURAL COMPETENCE

Specific terms relevant to cultural competence should be explored within the context of training. Specifically, a glossary of terms should be provided in training packets so that attendees can refer and recall pertinent information when necessary. Examples of key terms include the terms *stereotypes* and *cultural sensitivity*. If a staff member knows that **stereotypes** (as indicated in Chapter 4) are exaggerated beliefs or fixed ideas about a person and the term is taught within the context of a particular example that expresses how this process can impact the provision of services to an individual, negative attitudes and behaviors associated with the term may be avoided.

Additionally, understanding that the concept of **cultural sensitivity** refers to an awareness of and respect for a patient's cultural beliefs and values and understanding how to ensure that cultural sensitivity is implemented, by using scenarios presented in a training format, can be helpful in ensuring optimal, culturally competent care. Providing knowledge-based information is essential at all levels of healthcare and public health organizations because it brings key aspects of cultural competence to the forefront. The ultimate goal is to establish attitudes, behaviors, and practices that enable individuals, healthcare organizations, and public health entities to effectively serve culturally diverse communities.

Case Studies

Case studies can serve as tools to facilitate understanding by imparting information and putting key terms into practice. For example, consider the following case study:

> Lia, a 32-year-old woman from the Dominican Republic, is diagnosed with syphilis. She has been in the United States with her husband and four children for 3 years. She is pregnant and is afraid to tell her husband that she has the disease for fear that he will be angry with her. She speaks very limited English, and her primary language is Spanish. She knows a public health practitioner who works in her community at a local center that provides condoms and informational materials about sexually transmitted diseases in the community. Lia is reluctant to share her problem with the public health practitioner but nervously tries, although communication between the two of them is very poor because Lia is embarrassed that she does not speak English very well and is afraid to share her feelings. The public health practitioner learns from Lia that her husband is quite fluent in English and asks her if she

can bring him to the center so that they can discuss treatment options and provide him with condoms. Lia never returns a call to the public health practitioner after this request and does not speak to anyone else about the possibility of treatment.

This case provides great fodder for training because there are myriad issues involved. The first issue is that Lia is Spanish speaking and from the Dominican Republic. Consequently, culturally and linguistically, there are some differences that exist between the public health practitioner and Lia. Furthermore, there is a lack of cultural sensitivity exhibited by the public health practitioner because she is willing to use the husband of the client as an interpreter in an attempt to communicate without understanding a possible important nuance of Lia's culture. In the Dominican culture, the husband or oldest male is considered the head of the family and should be consulted regarding health-related decisions (Rundle, Carvalho, & Robinson, 2002). However, in matters of such a personal nature, bringing the husband in to talk and provide condoms may not be the best approach because most Dominicans are Roman Catholic and this may not be appropriate (Rundle et al.).

Additionally, the concerns that Lia has about sharing her illness with her husband are not being considered. Perhaps the best approach would be to use a trained interpreter to impart information to Lia and provide an informative brochure that is translated into Spanish that she can share with her husband, using her discretion and knowledge of how to best approach the subject with him.

Case studies are an excellent training tool for cultural competence. Through case studies, relevant terms can be shared and applied to actual or hypothetical scenarios.

KEY COMPONENTS OF CULTURAL COMPETENCE TRAINING

The key components of cultural competence training for healthcare organizations and public health entities include the following. First, overall objectives should be stated regarding what the training is intending to accomplish. Next, an overview should be provided of the importance of cultural competence, including a discussion of racial and ethnic disparities in health care and demographic changes in the United States (racially, ethnically, and linguistically). After this overview, relevant knowledge-based terminology pertinent to cultural competence should be defined, including terms such as ethnicity, race, culture, stereotyping, cultural sensitivity, cultural competence, linguistic competence, cultural nuances, and so on. As mentioned earlier, a glossary of terms should be provided in audience members' cultural competence training packets for review, consideration, and future use (see Appendix IV). An overview and detailed information regarding the minority groups in the United States, as identified by the Office of Management and Budget, should be provided, with a focus on the groups that are primarily served by the particular healthcare or public health organization. Determination of groups served should be based on demographic data that are collected about the patients/clients/customers the organization serves. Training should include relevant exercises and case studies involving role play and discussion on key issues pertaining to cultural competence and health care. Information should be provided regarding the proper use of interpreters, including who should be used (trained interpreters, either in person or by telephone) and who should not be used (family members, children, untrained interpreters, and bilingual staff). The use of the latter may lead to misinterpretations, inclusion of personal opinions in the interpretation process, and violation of confidentiality.

In addition, during training, organizational-level cultural competence should be discussed, including supportive policies and the need for commitment at every level of the organization, including the board of directors and top-level executives. Emphasis should be placed on the importance of diversity of the workforce, but the distinction between the terms diversity and cultural competence should also be emphasized. Participants should be informed that participation in training is an integral component of career development because having knowledge and insight regarding cultural competence is an enhancement for individuals at every level of the organization. Table 8-1 provides examples of modules and topics which may be included in cultural competence trainings.

EVALUATION OF CULTURAL COMPETENCE TRAINING

Because the primary purpose of cultural competence training sessions is to increase knowledge of multicultural factors that may impact the provision of healthcare services, to provide resources to assist in the implementation of a plan to institutionalize cultural competence throughout the organization, and to explore concepts pertaining to cultural and linguistic competence, all sessions should be evaluated to ensure that these objectives are accomplished. A systemized approach is necessary to accomplish evaluation. Primarily, an evaluation form should be provided after each training session, allowing responses in both a close-ended and open-ended format. The evaluation forms should be reviewed to determine whether the sessions met the intended goals and

Table 8-1 Sample Training with Modules

Training Format	
Administer cultural competence pretest	
Module I: Culture, race, and ethnicity	Review of the four largest minority groups: (1) African Americans, (2) Asians/Pacific Islanders, (3) Hispanic Americans, and (4) Native Americans
Module II: Cultural self-assessment	Attitudinal assessment tools (see appendices for assessment tools)
Module III: Cultural competence vs cultural proficiency: What is the difference?	• The need for a paradigm shift • Necessary skills • The Cultural Competence Continuum
Module IV: Overview of specific cultures (choose the predominant cultures served by the organization)	Example 1: African American and Caribbean culture and health • Historical perspective • Social support • The Tuskegee Syphilis Study • Case studies • Avoidance of stereotypes • The Caribbean (an overview)
Module V: Overview of specific cultures (choose the predominant cultures served by the organization)	Example 2: The Asian/Pacific Islander population • Immigration to the United States • Cultural standards • Belief in preventative medicine • Language barriers • Traditional medicine beliefs
Module VI: Overview of specific cultures (choose the predominant cultures served by the organization)	Example 3: The Hispanic population • Latino/Hispanic classification • Overview of Hispanics in the United States • Perceptions of health care • Traditional medicine beliefs • The culture of migrant farm workers
Module VII: Overview of specific cultures (choose the predominant cultures served by the organization)	Example 4: The Native American population • Federal tribes and land • The Indian Health Service • Language and cultural obstacles • Perceptions of health care • Traditional medicine beliefs
Module VIII: Elements of a culturally competent system of care	• Essential elements • Culturally and Linguistically Appropriate Services standards • Action plan
Administer cultural competence posttest	

whether participants have suggestions that may improve training or provide insight in terms of additional information that may be valuable. Information from the evaluations should be taken seriously, and training sessions should be modified or enhanced if participants have suggestions. Furthermore, customer satisfaction surveys should be modified to include specific questions pertaining to cultural competence based on information provided in the training sessions. Through customer satisfaction surveys, insight can be gleaned as to whether information from the training is being incorporated into the process of serving customers, and if not, retraining may be necessary. Evaluation should be a fluid and ongoing process, ensuring that the organization is maintaining a high level of cultural competence, identifying areas of strength and weakness, and continually providing education as needed.

CONCLUSIONS

Cultural competence training is needed in healthcare and public health organizations to ensure that the necessary requirements of diverse populations are met. This training should be part of an effort that also includes a diverse workforce and overall policies that support cultural competence efforts. Although it may be necessary to hire bilingual staff, use trained interpreters, hire multicultural vendors and contractors, and create marketing materials that are linguistically appropriate, it is imperative that steps are taken to ensure that the histories and cultures of populations are considered when services are provided. Hence, training is necessary to provide cross-cultural information at healthcare and public health organizations. All healthcare organizations and public health entities are different, with varying needs pertaining to cultural competence. Thus, evaluation methods should be designed to meet the organization's goals, but at the very least, they should include an evaluative survey tool and the inclusion of cultural competence questions into customer satisfaction surveys.

CHAPTER SUMMARY

In the United States, there is a disparity between the health status of White people and the health status of people of color, leading to poorer health outcomes for people of color. The United States has a history of social and economic discrimination of people of color, and healthcare disparities occur within the context of this history (Smedley, Stith, & Nelson, 2003). Therefore, cultural competence is necessary to inform individuals at every level of healthcare and public health organizations, including the board of directors, executives, staff, and providers, about these disparities and issues that are particularly important in serving diverse populations. A variety of training approaches, key components, and essential requirements exist to ensure success. All training should be evaluated through the use of a questionnaire with both close-ended and open-ended responses to get feedback so that training can be modified as necessary based on input from participants.

CHAPTER PROBLEMS

1. A healthcare organization decides to provide cultural competence training for providers because they have direct contact with customers. A decision is made that training is not needed for any other individuals at the organization, particularly those who are not clinicians. Is this the best approach? Why or why not?

2. A training session is provided at a public health organization on the need for linguistic competence when working in non-English-speaking communities. Upon completion of the training, staff are encouraged to contact the trainer if they have questions or feedback. What additional steps should the trainer take to acquire feedback from the participants? Why?

3. A CEO of a healthcare organization is working on the annual budget with the chief financial officer (CFO). A decision is made to include cultural competence training in the budget to occur at the beginning of the fiscal year. No other funds are allocated for additional training, other than the one time, because the CEO indicates that the training should be a one-shot deal that is comprehensive and thorough enough to ensure cultural competence for all. Will this be sufficient for the organization? Why or why not?

4. What are the key components of cultural competence training?

5. At the conclusion of a cultural competence training session at a healthcare organization, participants are provided with a binder including information from the training and a glossary of terms relevant to the subject matter. A staff member places the binder in her desk and does not look at the material again. How might the staff member use the glossary of terms, for example, to assist her with her day-to-day interactions with customers?

REFERENCES

Brathwaite, A. C., & Majumdar, B. (2006). Evaluation of a cultural competence education programme. *Journal of Advanced Nursing, 53*(4), 470–479.

Rundle, A., Carvalho, M., & Robinson, M. (2002). *Cultural competence in health care: A practical guide* (pp. 47–49). San Francisco: Jossey-Bass.

Smedley, B. D., Stith, A. Y., & Nelson, A. R. (Eds.). (2003). *Unequal treatment: Confronting racial and ethnic disparities in health care* (pp. 29–79). Washington, DC: The National Academies Press.

SUGGESTED READINGS

Dixon, M. (2006). *Strategies for cultural competency in Indian healthcare.* Washington, DC: American Public Health Association.

Fraker, D. (1999). *Cultural competence compendium.* Chicago: American Medical Association.

Gilbert, J. (Ed.). (2003). *A manager's guide to cultural competence education for health care professionals.* Woodland Hills, CA: The California Endowment.

Ring, J., Nyquist, J., & Mitchell, S. (2008). *Curriculum for culturally responsive health care: The step-by-step guide for cultural competence training.* Abingdon, United Kingdom: Radcliffe Publishing.

Wheeler, C., Jarvis, B., & Petty, R. (2001). Think unto others: The self destructive impact of negative racial stereotypes. *Journal of Experimental Psychology, 37*(2), 173–180.

Williamson, E., Stecchi, J., Allen, B., & Coppens, N. (1997). The development of culturally appropriate health education materials. *Journal of Nursing Staff Development, 13*(1), 19–23.

Culturally and Linguistically Appropriate Services Standards: An Overview

LEARNING OBJECTIVES

After reading this chapter, you should be able to:

- Discuss the Culturally and Linguistically Appropriate Services (CLAS) standards and their relevance to health services administration and public health.
- Understand how health service administrators can use these standards to develop an action plan and what should be included.
- Explain why qualitative research is an effective approach for evaluating cultural competence training necessary to provide staff with information about CLAS.

KEY TERMS

CLAS standards	Wisdom of crowds

INTRODUCTION

This chapter will focus exclusively on the Culturally and Linguistically Appropriate Services (CLAS) standards in health care as an administrative initiative. These standards were developed by the Office of Minority Health (OMH), US Department of Health and Human Services (US DHHS), and were released in December 2000 (OMH, US DHHS, 2000) and include guidelines, recommendations, and mandates, with the potential to create a more consistent way of looking at culture in terms of health across the country. The 14 standards will be reviewed, emphasizing how they are grouped based on the following three themes: Culturally Competent Care (standards 1–3), Language Access Services (standards 4–7), and Organizational Supports for Cultural Competence (standards 8–14). This chapter also focuses on how health service administrators can use these standards to develop action plans that include assessment, education, implementation, reassessment, and validation of cultural competence within health service organizations. The importance of qualitative research as an evaluative mechanism for cultural competence will also be explored.

CULTURALLY AND LINGUISTICALLY APPROPRIATE STANDARDS

The purpose of the **CLAS standards** is to address the inequities that exist in the provision of health care and to make services more responsive to the individual needs, on a cultural and linguistic basis, of patients/clients/consumers served. The ultimate goal of the CLAS national standards is to improve the health of all who seek care in the United States through the elimination of racial and ethnic health disparities, which is an enormous challenge. Key features of the CLAS standards are as follows:

- Provide a common understanding and consistent definitions of culturally and linguistically appropriate services in health care
- Offer a practical framework for the implementation of services and organizational structures that can help healthcare organizations and providers be responsive to the cultural and linguistic issues presented by diverse populations

The CLAS standards (Table 9-1) were initially derived from an analysis of current practices and policies on cultural competence and shaped by the experiences and expertise of healthcare organizations, policymakers, and consumers; they were developed over a 3-year period based on input from a number of sources, as sponsored by the OMH, US DHHS. Written documents of both technical and policy literature were reviewed. Technical literature, including reports on research studies, and philosophical and disciplinary papers served as background materials for the cultural and linguistic competence elements of the standards. The policy literature included legal reports, federal and state statutory and regulatory documents, accreditation guidelines, reports on cultural competence standards or measures, and provider contract documents from select state-managed care providers.

Table 9-1 Culturally and Linguistically Appropriate Services (CLAS) Standards

Themes	Standards
Culturally Competent Care (standards 1–3)	1. Healthcare organizations should ensure that patients/consumers receive from all staff members, effective, understandable, and respectful care that is provided in a manner compatible with their cultural beliefs and practices and preferred languages.
	2. Healthcare organizations should implement strategies to recruit, retain, and promote at all levels of the organization a diverse staff and leadership that are representative of the demographic characteristics of the service area.
	3. Healthcare organizations should ensure that staff at all levels and across all disciplines receive ongoing education and training in culturally and linguistically appropriate service delivery.
Language Access Services (standards 4–7)	4. Healthcare organizations must offer and provide language assistance services, including bilingual staff and interpreter services, at no cost to each patient/consumer with limited English proficiency at all points of contact, in a timely manner during all hours of operation.
	5. Healthcare organizations must provide to patients/consumers in their preferred language both verbal offers and written notices informing them of their right to receive language assistance services.
	6. Healthcare organizations must assure the competence of language assistance provided to limited English patients/consumers by interpreters and bilingual staff. Family and friends should not be used to provide interpretation services (except on request by the patient/consumer).
	7. Healthcare organizations must make available easily understood patient-related materials and post signage in the languages of the commonly encountered groups and/or groups represented in the service area.
Organizational Supports for Cultural Competence (standards 8–14)	8. Healthcare organizations should develop, implement, and promote a written strategic plan that outlines clear goals, policies, operational plans, and management accountability/oversight mechanisms to provide culturally and linguistically appropriate services.
	9. Healthcare organizations should conduct initial and ongoing organizational self-assessments of CLAS-related activities and are encouraged to integrate cultural and linguistic competence–related measures into their internal audits, performance improvement programs, patient satisfaction assessments, and outcomes-based evaluations.
	10. Healthcare organizations should ensure that data on the individual patient's/consumer's race, ethnicity, and spoken and written language are collected in health records, integrated into the organization's management information systems, and periodically updated.

(continued)

Table 9-1 *(Continued)*

Themes	Standards
	11. Healthcare organizations should maintain a current demographic, cultural, and epidemiologic profile for the community as well as a needs assessment to accurately plan for and implement services that respond to the cultural and linguistic characteristics of the service area.
	12. Healthcare organizations should develop participatory, collaborative partnerships with communities and utilize a variety of formal and informal mechanisms to facilitate community and patient/consumer involvement in designing and implementing CLAS-related activities.
	13. Healthcare organizations should ensure that conflict and grievance resolution processes are culturally and linguistically sensitive and capable of identifying, preventing, and resolving cross-cultural conflicts or complaints by patients/consumers.
	14. Healthcare organizations are encouraged to regularly make available to the public information about their progress and successful innovations in implementing the CLAS standards and to provide public notice in their communities about the availability of this information.

Source: Data from US Department of Health and Human Services. (2001). Cultural competency part II. *Closing the Gap*, February/March, 3.

The standards are primarily aimed at healthcare organizations, particularly hospitals, but are also relevant for other types of organizations, including public health entities. The standards are organized per three themes, as delineated in Table 9-1, which are:

- Culturally Competent Care (standards 1–3)
- Language Access Services (standards 4–7)
- Organizational Supports for Cultural Competence (standards 8–14)

Within this structure, there are three types of standards of varying severity. These are mandates, guidelines, and recommendations. CLAS mandates are current federal requirements for all recipients of federal funds and are expanded upon in standards 4, 5, and 6. CLAS guidelines are recommendations by the OMH for adoption as mandates by federal, state, and national accrediting agencies and are represented by standards 1, 2, 3, 8, 9, 10, 11, 12, and 13. Standard 14 is a recommendation by the OMH for voluntary implementation by organizations.

THE NEED FOR CLAS STANDARDS AND ACTION PLANS FOR ADMINISTRATORS

Even without mandates and standards, it should be the case, in today's society, that every member of American society is treated with respect and consideration of their cultural beliefs and is provided with appropriately interpreted communication. Nevertheless, to ensure that this occurs, administrators and public health practitioners can develop and implement action plans that include assessment, education, implementation, ongoing reassessment, and validation of CLAS across their organizations. In pursuing such an action plan, first a series of questions should be asked; these are as follows:

1. What cultural issues or challenges should the organization begin addressing now?
2. What are the barriers to addressing these issues?
3. What are the available resources and supports to begin and implement the process?
4. How can management at various levels of the organization facilitate change in cultural attitudes, behaviors, and values?
5. How prepared is this organization to effectively respond to the cultural practices and nuances of patients/clients/customers?

Once these questions have been reviewed, analyzed, and answered, the next step is to begin the organization of cultural competence efforts at the organization. An initial step should be the identification of interpretation services to address linguistic competence issues.

Additionally, administrators should ensure that patients/clients/customers are provided with appropriately translated written materials and signage in the languages of the predominant groups served by the organization. Therefore, within the actual facilities where patients/clients/customers are served, projects should ensue that there is of multilingual signage, visual affirmations, and translation of brochures and important documents to be distributed to patients. Hence, a review of demographic data should be undertaken to provide insight into the prevalent languages spoken by patients/clients/customers who use the facility. Simultaneously, workforce diversity should be reviewed with the goal of ensuring that the workforce is appropriately diverse. A cultural competence plan is always evolving, and as the demographics of the community change, efforts toward updates must also take place. The health services or public health organization should never be caught off guard in terms of cultural competence. Ensuring that a robust continuous improvement plan is in place will serve the organization well. Web sites of healthcare and public health organizations should include pages that specifically focus on and visually affirm the cultural groups served and that are available for community and staff perusal. The Internet can also be used as an opportunity for staff to find information and insight regarding cultural competence.

To prompt cultural competence efforts, administrators and public health practitioners must ensure that staff education takes place, including the provision of information regarding the cultural norms of the predominant groups served by the organization, presentations by experts regarding universal communication techniques across cultures, and a complete overview of the CLAS standards. There are various types of learning that should be considered in the training process. As stated by Cox (2001), three types of learning that should be considered are:

(1) consciousness raising,
(2) providing new information about diverse groups, and
(3) actions to promote diversity information. (p. 9)

Cox (2001) further states, in terms of training, "arrange for sequenced events rather than one day marathons. Use a variety of teaching tools, videos, small-group discussion, mini lectures" (p. 9). This training must be evaluated carefully to ensure efficacy. Quantitative and qualitative approaches can be used, but qualitative research has proven to be an effective approach to evaluate cultural competence training programs.

QUALITATIVE RESEARCH

Qualitative health research, with respect to cultural competence training, has emerged as an acceptable means of analysis of programs and the content absorbed by the participants. Focus groups, originally based in the social sciences, are now being used across a wide cross section of fields such as education, communication studies, political science, and public health. With respect to public health, focus groups are used to develop and evaluate programs (Colucci, 2007). For instance, research that has been conducted using qualitative approaches includes studies on immigration issues with second-generation Filipino youth, on health concerns and access to health care of young people living in rural and urban Australia, on men and their experience with depression, on the social construction of sexually transmitted infections in South African communities, and on the underlying attitude toward tuberculosis and its context in the Democratic Republic of Congo (Colucci).

When reviewing focus groups from a healthcare setting, there are many advantages that make the group setting ideal in an effort to glean critical information. For example, a group setting will allow a moderator to ask a particular question in an effort to make the group "do" something and answer questions in a more active way. This action, while perhaps viewed by some as "psychological tricks or stimulus," can yield results that may not have been formally known in the particular community or group. For instance, individuals who will not normally voice an opinion contrary to their familial social structure are more likely to be vocal in a group setting moderated by a member of the same sex. Hypothetically speaking, we could make this inference about Asian women or women from the Middle East, for example, for whom a more male-dominated society and culture demand a specific level of deference to the patriarchal system.

Hence, qualitative research is a valuable in healthcare cultural competence training evaluation because it allows an in-depth review of programs and the effectiveness of learning by the participants. For example, in a study conducted in Canada, the effectiveness of cultural competence training was measured, based on a quantitative and qualitative process, to determine the overall effectiveness and whether there were any increases in the level of competence by the participants. Participants were separated into different groups and given incentives to participate in the surveys and focus group studies; the data were then measured and compared (Braithwaite & Majumdar, 2006). Prior to the study, a baseline level of knowledge was determined by a standardized test. After training, a standardized test was administered, and the demographic and baseline data were analyzed statistically. Qualitatively, data were obtained through focus groups and by open-ended questions. When the analysis was complete, the quantitative results were confirmed by the qualitative results of the team. Although most participants did report on their surveys that there was an increase in cultural knowledge, the majority of participants also noted that the effectiveness of the program was successful due to the other factors that were discussed during the focus group sessions. For instance, the peers shared specifically what they learned and further knowledge gained during and after training sessions and provided insight into their consultations with one another during and after the sessions. This study indicated that quantitative studies can often be limited by the extent of the tool used to gather information. In contrast, qualitative research lends to collective predictions or a collaborative filter known as **wisdom of crowds**. Consequently, to evaluate cultural competence training, qualitative insight from members of groups who were participants can provide useful, detailed, and comprehensive information.

Additionally, beyond the training and evaluation processes, health service administrators and public health officials should ensure that contractors and vendors serving the organization and its constituents are also culturally competent. Upon review of their proposals or requests to provide services to organizations, cultural competence skills and capabilities should be considered, along with the primary services the contractors and vendors intend to provide. Linguistic competence and the diversification of their staff should be considered to ensure that all organizations that interface with health service organizations and public health entities are operating from the same vantage point.

CONCLUSIONS

Diversity in the United States is here to stay and increasing. As a result, it is imperative that healthcare organizations embrace this fact and work toward ensuring culturally appropriate services for all patients/clients/customers. The purpose of the OMH's national CLAS standards is to facilitate the process of ensuring optimal services to all, regardless of race, ethnicity, culture, or language(s) spoken. These standards attempt to address the potential inequities that exist, culturally and linguistically, in the provision of health care with the goal of making healthcare services responsive to the needs of all people served. The ultimate aim of the CLAS standards is to improve health through the elimination of racial and ethnic disparities. Consequently, healthcare administrators have the responsibility of leading their organizations to meet the CLAS standards. The goal of healthcare organizations should ultimately be to ensure systems, processes, and a workforce whose primary aim is to deliver excellent care with maximum efficiency to all patients/clients/customers. This must be accomplished without bias, and thus, race, ethnicity, culture, and primary language spoken should not be factors in determining whether or not individuals receive quality care. All individuals should receive optimal service as ensured by health service administrators and public health practitioners.

CHAPTER SUMMARY

The CLAS standards serve to ensure that all members of society will have equal provision of health services. The real success of CLAS will be when such standards are no longer needed, and individuals will be respected and provided with equal access to healthcare services that are delivered within the scope of appropriate linguistic services and consideration of cultural norms. Healthcare organizations are responsible for recognizing the value of considering and understanding cultural norms in the provision of services to people from different cultural backgrounds. Within the context of the action plan to implement CLAS, it should be understood that cultural competence is not a "stand-alone" outcome, but must be integrated into the entire organization. Administrators must be willing to allocate and re-allocate resources to support program initiatives and develop institutional benchmarks and reward successes (Institute of Medicine, 2001). Hence, the role of leadership is extremely important to any cultural competence action plan. The support of leadership is required to recognize, prioritize, and drive efforts that establish polices and procedures that improve care to better meet the needs of diverse populations.

CHAPTER PROBLEMS

1. Standards 4–7 of the CLAS standards are designed to ensure organizational support for cultural competence. Is this an accurate statement? Explain.
2. An administrator of a healthcare facility decides that there is a need to proceed with an action plan to implement the CLAS standards. What initial questions should he ask and acquire answers to before beginning the process?
3. Evaluation of training is essential to ensure effectiveness. The quality assurance director at a healthcare facility advises the chief executive officer that the only approach to doing so is quantitative research using a close-ended survey before and after each training session. What other approach should be considered, and what type of information may be acquired in doing so?
4. What is the purpose of the CLAS standards, and why are they relevant to health care today?
5. A customer enters a public health facility to acquire information about swine flu and the potential impact of the influenza. She speaks Creole and is lost in the building. Finally, she is able to locate someone who is able to ascertain that she is in need of information about swine flu. She is given a brochure that is written in English. She leaves the facility feeling nervous and unable to read the brochure she received. Per the CLAS standards, what should have been done to ensure that the customer was served effectively?

REFERENCES

Braithwaite, A., & Majumdar, B. (2006). Evaluation of a cultural competence education programme. *Journal of Advanced Nursing, 53*(4), 470–479.
Colucci, E. (2007). Focus groups can be fun: The use of activity-oriented questions in focus group discussions. *Qualitative Health Research, 17*(10), 1422–1433.

Cox, T., Jr. (2001). *Creating the multicultural organization: A strategy for capturing the power of diversity*. San Francisco: John Wiley & Sons.

Institute of Medicine. (2001). *Crossing the quality chasm: A new health system for the 21st century: Formulating new rules to redesign and improve care*. Washington, DC: National Academies Press.

Office of Minority Health, US Department of Health and Human Services. (2000). National standards on Culturally and Linguistically Appropriate Services (CLAS) in health care. *Federal Register, 65*(247), 80865–80879.

SUGGESTED READINGS

Gorrin, S., Arnold, J., & Green, L. (2006). *Health promotion and practice*. San Francisco: Jossey-Bass.

Laveist, T. (2005). *Minority populations and health: An introduction to health disparities in the U.S.* San Francisco: Jossey-Bass.

Longest, B. (2004). *Managing health programs and projects*. San Francisco: Jossey Bass.

Zaza, S. (2005). *The guide to community preventive services: What works to promote health? Task Force on Community Preventive Services*. New York: Oxford University Press.

Chapter 10

The Ultimate Challenge: Educational and Institutional Considerations

LEARNING OBJECTIVES

After reading this chapter, you should be able to:

- Understand current accreditation requirements for healthcare organizations.
- Delineate key accrediting organizations and their requirements/perspectives on cultural competence.
- Recognize the importance of necessary educational initiatives in terms of healthcare administration and public health.

┌─ **KEY TERMS** ───

Agency for Healthcare Research and Quality (AHRQ)

American Medical Association (AMA)

Commission on Accreditation of Healthcare Management Education (CAHME)

Council on Education for Public Health (CEPH)

Institute of Medicine (IOM)

The Joint Commission

Sullivan Commission

└──

INTRODUCTION

This chapter focuses on current accreditation requirements for healthcare organizations relevant to cultural competence. Insight regarding specific accrediting organizations and advisory organizations, such as the

Council on Education for Public Health (CEPH), the American Medical Association (AMA), the Commission on Accreditation of Healthcare Management Education (CAHME), and The Joint Commission, and their requirements/perspectives on cultural competence will be provided in a brief, introductory format. Key reports and studies will be highlighted, including those from the Institute of Medicine (IOM), the Agency for Healthcare Research and Quality (AHRQ), and the Sullivan Commission. Recommendations are also made regarding the necessary educational requirements that should be considered in terms of healthcare administration and public health education to increase cultural competence levels. A challenge will be posed to health service administrators and public health practitioners to take steps to move cultural competence forward, highlighting concrete ideas and possibilities that are within reach. It is important to note that this chapter merely provides an overview of accrediting and advisory organizations and their initiatives in terms of cultural competence.

THE AMERICAN MEDICAL ASSOCIATION

According to the AMA's Web site (www.ama-assn.org/), individuals are asked to join the organization for the following reasons:

> The AMA impacts the daily work of **all** physicians, residents, fellow and medical students in the U.S. In recent years, we've tackled crucial topics like medical liability, clinical quality, managed care, patient safety, Medicare billing and payment, medical education debt and more.

Furthermore, the AMA is quite involved in providing input regarding medical school curricula. According to Champaneria and Axtell (2004), medical students are benefitting from cross-cultural exchanges and cultural competence training, although there are limited outcome data from the training. It is safe to say that although the AMA considers the topic of cultural competence important, the organization's primary concern, in terms of minorities, is health disparities. The **AMA** is not an accrediting organization per se, but provides insight and information regarding the medical field and support for physicians. AMA also has a public health focus that entails promoting healthy lifestyles, providing resources for health professionals, and serving as a center for public health preparedness, disaster response, and vaccination resources. In general, it works to advance quality improvement in patient care.

THE COMMISSION ON ACCREDITATION OF HEALTHCARE MANAGEMENT EDUCATION

The **CAHME** is an accrediting body that sets criteria regarding healthcare management. Essentially, the organization works closely with educational programs to ensure that they are improving. CAHME has a specific criterion that programs must meet, number IIIB1 (item 5), that states the following: "Mobilizing community action to address health problems including cultural competence" (CAHME, n.d.) This organization was actually initiated by healthcare management programs in an effort to foster peer review and self-management and focuses only on healthcare management at the graduate level (master's degree programs). Given that cultural competence is mentioned in its framework for accreditation, it is expected that the organization considers it as part of its primary focus. CAHME also emphasizes diversity, which has been established in this text as a separate but equally important requirement, beyond cultural competence, for health services administrations and public health organizations.

THE JOINT COMMISSION

The Joint Commission, as mentioned in Chapter 6, is the accrediting body for healthcare organizations, including hospitals, community health centers, and other types of healthcare facilities. In terms of cultural competence, The Joint Commission recognizes the importance of culturally competent care and has been doing so since 2004. In Chapter 6, standards that are relevant to cultural competence are discussed. Here, we will discuss a research study that The Joint Commission implemented exploring cultural competence. The Joint Commission, with funding from the California Endowment, initiated a cross-sectional language study entitled *Hospitals, Language, and Culture: A Snapshot of the Nation* (HLC). The HLC studied 60 hospitals across the country to ascertain how they provide culturally and linguistically competent care to diverse populations (The Joint Commission, 2009). The research was based on the fact that, as indicated throughout this text, demographics in the United States have changed, leading to more US residents who are foreign born and who do not speak English. The HLC study was aimed at conducting research around this issue.

The HLC report was released in April 2008 and essentially concludes that there is no one-size-fits-all solution and that each organization has to develop its own approach to meet the needs of its patients/clients/customers. The report also advises developing a cultural competence plan akin to a business plan, as mentioned earlier in this text (see Appendix VI for a sample cultural competence plan). The key recommendations from this report (Wilson-Stronks, Lee, Cordero, Kopp, & Galvez, 2008) are as follows:

- Identify the needs of the patient population being served and assess how well these needs are being met through current systems.
- Bring people across the organization together to explore cultural and language issues by sharing experiences, evaluating current practices, discussing barriers, and identifying gaps.
- Make assessment, monitoring, and evaluation of cultural and language needs and services a continuous process.

This report includes a self-assessment tool that organizations can use to initiate discussions about the needs, resources, and goals for providing the highest quality care to every patient served.

THE COUNCIL ON EDUCATION FOR PUBLIC HEALTH

The **CEPH** is an organization that accredits institutions that prepare graduates for public health practice. The organization accredits public health schools and programs based on a number of specific criteria that must be met. Schools and programs must conduct a comprehensive self-study, provide required documentation, and undergo a site visit. CEPH focuses intently on diversity in that one of the criteria requires the recruitment, retention, and promotion of diverse faculty regardless of race, age, gender, disability, sexual orientation, religion, or national origin. Per CEPH criteria, diversity is also required in terms of the student population. Diversity and cultural competence are two distinctly different concepts, and therefore, criteria related to diversity do not necessarily address cultural competence. Although CEPH seeks evidence of diversity, the organization should develop criteria that are specific to cultural competence based on the definition of the term and perhaps in adherence to the Culturally and Linguistically Appropriate Services (CLAS) healthcare standards modified to address requirements for students and faculty. Perhaps the criteria could require evidence that the standards are being taught, that students are receiving training in cultural competence, and that faculty are aptly trained to teach cultural competence.

THE INSTITUTE OF MEDICINE

The **IOM** is a component of the National Academy of Sciences, and its purpose is to advise the nation about health, biomedical science, and medicine. IOM has produced a number of significant and timely reports primarily focusing on health disparities. Inherent in the discussion of healthcare disparities is the need for cultural competence because the lack of cultural competence contributes to the problem of the gap between the health status of minorities and Whites, where Whites fare better. A particularly important report was titled *Unequal Treatment: Confronting Racial and Ethnic Disparities in Health Care* (Smedley, Stith, & Nelson, 2002). This report, along with others, made it clear that minority groups do not receive equal treatment in terms of care and hence cultural competence is needed. Advice such as this is important in ensuring that the nation remains focused on meeting the needs of the various minority groups in the United States. Although the IOM is not an accrediting body, the advice that it provides in its numerous reports with ensuing recommendations is invaluable in continuously sounding the alarm regarding the need for culturally competent care.

THE AGENCY FOR HEALTHCARE RESEARCH AND QUALITY

The **AHRQ** is 1 of 12 agencies within the Department of Health and Human Services (DHHS). Its mission is to improve the quality, safety, efficiency, and effectiveness of health care for all Americans. In 2004, the AHRQ produced a report entitled *Setting the Agenda for Research on Cultural Competence in Healthcare* (Fortier & Bishop, 2004). The purpose of the research project was to look at the impact cultural competence interventions have on the delivery of health care and health outcomes and investigate the opportunities and barriers that affect how further research in this area might be conducted. The result of the study was an indication that further efforts are needed to research the efficacy of cultural competence due to problems such as lack of standardized definitions of interventions and standardized evaluative measures (Fortier & Bishop). Consequently, it appears that the value of AHRQ, in terms of cultural competence, is to provide research on the matter in line with its mission of enhancing health care for all.

THE SULLIVAN COMMISSION

Under the leadership of Dr. Louis W. Sullivan, former US Secretary of Health and Human Services, and Dr. Lonnie R. Bristow, former President of the American Medical Association, the Sullivan Alliance to Transform America's Health Professions was established and is known as the **Sullivan Commission**. The Sullivan Commission is primarily a diversity initiative and attempts to reduce racial and ethnic disparities through increasing diversity in the health professions. Therefore, the commission has a tangential goal of cultural competence because, as mentioned previously, diversity initiatives are not the same as cultural competence efforts. However, given that one of the goals of cultural competence is to reduce health disparities, the Sullivan Commission is worthy of serious consideration in this context. In a report entitled *Missing Persons: Minorities in the Health Professions*, the Sullivan Commission (2004) makes recommendations that directly include cultural competence as a complementary strategy for increasing diversity and consider it as an initiative that would be more apt to be embraced by minority health professionals. The report also recommends cultural competence training for healthcare professionals and includes it as part of organizational strategic plans.

NECESSARY EDUCATIONAL REQUIREMENTS

Recommendations concerning educational requirements for students will perhaps be useful and should be considered in terms of health service administration and public health education in an effort to increase cultural competence levels. The first recommendation is to ensure that students are provided with the CLAS standards, with a full overview and explanation of each. Once this is accomplished, students should be given an explanation as to why cultural competence is needed, with an emphasis on the reduction of health disparities between minorities and Whites and the provision of efficacious services without cultural and linguistic barriers. Students should also be supplied with comprehensive literature on these issues and comparative health data on the various minority groups and Whites. Furthermore, students should be informed that the demographics are changing in the United States at significant rates and that there is a growing population with limited English proficiency. Students should also understand that language obstacles/barriers can lead to patients/clients/customers avoiding care because the process is too challenging.

Many of the terms associated with cultural competence are complex and require explanation. Hence, a glossary of key terms relevant to cultural competence, as provided in this text (see Appendix IV), should be explored in depth so that students understand the difference between cultural competence and diversity and learn the definitions for terms related to cultural competence, such as socioeconomic status, ethnicity, religion, stereotypes, cultural sensitivity, and so on. Students should experience the same types of training sessions as healthcare professionals, as indicated in Table 8-2, with varying modules to provide insight into some of the specifics of cultural competence. The Assumption Exercise, which is discussed in Chapter 5, should also be part of their training so that students understand the inherent problems involved with making assumptions about individuals. Case studies that are germane to minority groups should also be reviewed so that students can grasp cultural nuances and differences within and between cultures and begin to formulate ideas on how to handle various scenarios that warrant culturally competent skill sets. Students should also learn about the importance of translation (written word) and interpretation (spoken word) for patients/clients/customers with limited English proficiency and become familiar with language services that may be available for utilization in health service and public health organizations. Beyond practical matters, health service administration and public health students should also learn about the need for cultural competence organizational policies and the incorporation of cultural competence into directive strategies of the organization, including development of cultural competence action plans.

Ultimately, these recommendations should prepare students to work in a culturally competent health service administration and public health workforce, with a diverse management team, and should qualify them to work with patients/clients/customers from various cultures and that speak different languages. Students should have insight into how to develop personnel policies that are supportive of cultural competence and should look to work for organizations that offer ongoing training and career development regarding cultural competence. Within the context of their curriculum, students should also experience cultural competence assessment to determine where they fit on the Cultural Competence Continuum, to determine areas of weakness, and to identify attitudinal concerns that may need to be adjusted prior to graduating from their health service administration or public health programs. Students need to be fully aware that when working with culturally diverse populations, visual affirmation is necessary in terms of marketing materials and linguistically appropriate education materials because cultural competence is a business goal, as well as an altruistic goal. Cultural competence is a process that requires continuous evaluation; therefore, students should learn evaluative techniques during their educational training so that they are prepared to determine whether cultural competence programs in their work environments, after acquiring their degrees, are effective.

CHALLENGING HEALTH SERVICE ADMINISTRATORS AND PUBLIC HEALTH PRACTITIONERS

The challenge for health service administrators and public health practitioners is to move cultural competence forward. One way this can be done is by enhancing educational curriculums to include cultural competence information. Moreover, it is important to recognize that cultural competence is not only about the people receiving services but also about those providing the services. Cultural competence lends to the growth of individuals, collective groups, and organizations. It is an ongoing learning process because culture evolves; it is not static. Demographics will continue to change, and organizations need to maintain a level of fluidity to adapt to the needs of their patients/clients/customers. Health service administrators and public health practitioners should take on the challenge of identifying where their organization is on the Cultural Competence Continuum and determine areas of improvement that will make a difference in serving patients/clients/customers. Health service and public health organizations should be physically inviting for the people they are designed to serve, and patients/clients/customers should be culturally affirmed when they seek services. Diversification has been and continues to be a primary concern for health service and public health organizations. However, the challenge now is to continue to diversify public health organizations and also ensure cultural competence within the organizations. Perhaps by reviewing the information in this text, students will have a greater understanding of the need for cultural competence and take on the challenge of carrying this effort forward indefinitely.

CONCLUSIONS

Accrediting organizations relevant to public health and health services organizations, programs, and schools are embracing the notions of diversity and cultural competence and moving toward standards and criteria to ensure the provision of efficacious service and comprehensive learning experiences for students. Some of these entities have further to go than others because diversity is still at the forefront, without processes in place enabling cultural competence efforts. Educational institutions that offer degrees in public health and health services administration will serve their students optimally by providing cultural competence training and education because the rapid demographic changes in American society are leading to more individuals seeking services who have limited English proficiency and who are from diverse culture groups.

CHAPTER SUMMARY

As organizations move toward meeting accreditation requirements pertaining to diversity and cultural competence, challenges emerge. One of these challenges is that accrediting institutions, particularly those involved in public health and health services administration, must rise to the occasion of recognizing the unique needs of individuals from various cultural groups and require that the organizations they accredit and advise are culturally competent. On a positive note, organizations such as the AMA, CAHME, CEPH, The Joint Commission, IOM, AHRQ, and Sullivan Commission are recognizing the need for cultural competence and moving their organizations toward advising, accrediting, conducting research on, and generally emphasizing the need for cultural competence. To that end, curricula need to be enhanced to ensure that public health and health service administration students are not being short changed because they lack information and training regarding cultural competence. Health service administrators and public health practitioners must be challenged to move cultural competence forward within their organizations. Cultural competence is important to people who are both receiving services and providing services and leads to growth of all.

CHAPTER PROBLEMS

1. A student is considering a master's degree in public health and is reviewing the curricula of various schools to make her final selection. In terms of cultural competence, what should she be looking for in her course options?
2. What are the AMA, CAHME, The Joint Commission, Sullivan Commission, AHRQ, CEPH, and IOM? What specifically is their relevance to cultural competence, if any?
3. Who started the Sullivan Commission, and what is the Commission's primary area of focus?
4. There are challenges that public health practitioners and health services administrators should be focusing on in terms of cultural competence. List two recommendations that they may want to consider.
5. What is limited English proficiency, and how might it serve as a problem for a person seeking health services?

REFERENCES

Commission on Accreditation of Healthcare Management Education. (n.d.), Candidacy Handbook, 22.

Champaneria, M. C., & Axtell, S. (2004). Cultural competence training in US medical schools. *Journal of the American Medical Association, 291*(17), 2142.

Fortier, J., & Bishop, D. (2004). *Setting the agenda for research on cultural competence in health care.* Rockville, MD: Agency for Healthcare Research and Quality.

Smedley, B. D., Stith, A. Y., & Nelson, A. R. (Eds.). (2002). *Unequal treatment: Confronting racial and ethnic disparities in health care.* Washington, DC: The National Academies Press.

Sullivan Commission. (2004). *Missing persons: Minorities in the health professions.* Battle Creek, MI: W.K. Kellog Foundation.

The Joint Commission. (2009). *Facts about the Hospitals, Language and Culture: A Snapshot of the Nations HLC study.* Retrieved April 2009, from http://www.jointcommission .org/AboutUs/Fact_Sheets/facts_hlc.htm.

Wilson-Stronks, A., Lee, K. K., Cordero, C. L., Kopp, A. L., & Galvez, E. (2008). *One size does not fit all: Meeting the health care needs of diverse populations.* Oakbrook Terrace, IL: The Joint Commission.

Suggested Readings

Institute of Medicine. (1994). *Balancing the scales of opportunity: Ensuring racial and ethnic diversity in the health professions.* Washington, DC: The National Academies Press.

Jones, C. P. (2001). Invited commentary: Race, racism, and the practice of epidemiology. *American Journal of Epidemiology, 154*(4), 299–304.

Krieger, N. (2001). The ostrich, the albatross, and public health: An ecosocial perspective—Or why an explicit focus on health consequences of discrimination and deprivation is vital for good science and public health practice. *Public Health Reports, 116*(5), 419–423.

Krieger, N. (2003). Does racism harm health? Did child abuse exist before 1962? On explicit questions, critical science, and current controversies: An ecosocial perspective. *American Journal of Public Health, 93*(2), 194–199.

Nazroo, J. Y. (2003). The structuring of ethnic inequalities in health: Economic position, racial discrimination, and racism. *American Journal of Public Health, 93*(2), 277–284.

Smith, D. B. (1999). *Health care divided: Race and healing a nation.* Ann Arbor, MI: University of Michigan Press.

Chapter 11

Cultural Competence and Women of Color

LEARNING OBJECTIVES

After reading this chapter, you should be able to:

- Discuss the relationship between health disparities and poverty, based on an example of teenage pregnancy among African American girls in Dade County, Florida.

- List culturally competent steps that will serve as positive additions to efforts to decrease teenage pregnancy among girls from diverse populations.

- Explain why the examples of culturally competent approaches are relevant to other public health concerns beyond teenage pregnancy.

- Identify linguistically appropriate approaches that are helpful in serving diverse communities.

- Provide insight regarding experiences unique to a special population, namely, women, in terms of healthcare administration and public health.

KEY TERMS

Gender	Simultaneous oppression
Interpretation	Translation
Middle passage	

INTRODUCTION

This chapter provides insight, through the review of an article published in the *Harvard Journal of Minority Public Health* entitled "Teenage Pregnancy and Poverty Among Black Teenagers" (Rose, 1998) and a further discussion of women of color in general, into important perspectives that should be considered regarding culture and other factors when providing health care. In previous chapters, the need for cultural competence has been established. Health disparities have also been discussed. Here, the aim is to show that lack of cultural competence can lead to the failure to understand pressing problems in American society, germane to health care and public health, and how incorrect conclusions and assumptions may be made about a group of individuals as a result. Furthermore, this chapter explores a special population in terms of health care in America, namely, women of color. The aforementioned article will serve as one example, and a discussion will ensue related to the unique needs and concerns of women from varying racial and ethnic groups, illustrated by case studies, in terms of health services administration and public health.

NEEDS ASSESSMENT

Teenage pregnancy was explored in depth by the author of this text in an article published in the *Harvard Journal of Minority Public Health* by reviewing the highlights of a needs assessment conducted by the South Florida Perinatal Healthy Start Coalition of Dade County (Figure 11-1).

Although the needs assessment was conducted in 1994, the conclusions of the study remain timely and are as follows:

- Poverty is a major contributing factor to teenage pregnancy, particularly among Black/African American girls.
- Programs focusing on economic assistance that foster independence for teenage, at-risk Black/African American girls are necessary.
- Sexual relations, pregnancy, and having children may be seen, by some teenagers who are poor, as one of the few lifestyle options that give them direction and a sense of purpose.
- Teenagers who feel a sense of helplessness in their lives as a result of poverty and who have few educational goals tend to use contraception less effectively.

Because teenage pregnancy is clearly a public health concern that seemingly occurs in greater numbers among young women of color compared with the mainstream population, the topic begs for understanding and

The Relationship Between Teenage Pregnancy and Poverty Among Black Teenagers

Revelations of a Dade County, Florida, Needs Assessment

by Patti R. Rose, EdD. MPH, Nova Southeastern University

Abstract

The South Florida Perinatal Healthy Start Coalition of Dade County, Florida conducted a county-wide maternal and infant health care needs assessment in 1994. The purpose of this paper is to highlight the findings of this needs assessment in relationship to teenage pregnancy and to provide insight into some of the findings, particularly those related to black teenage girls. The needs assessment indicates that teenage pregnancy occurs across all race/ethnic groups but that the problem is disproportionately high among black teenagers in Dade County. Certain factors relating to teenage pregnancy are considered in terms of demographic data revealed as a result of the needs assessment. Issues which need to be addressed in order to reduce the occurrence of teenage pregnancy are also explored.

Introduction

According to Healthy People 2000, the health objectives for the nation include a reduction in the proportion of adolescents engaging in sexual intercourse. Teenage pregnancy is increasingly becoming an area of focus for public health policy in the United States. There are over 13 million sexually active teenagers in this country.[1,4]

Patti R. Rose, EdD, MPH is an Assistant Professor of Public Health at Nova Southeastern University's Public Health Program in Fort Lauderdale, Florida.

Each year over 13 million girls under the age of 19 become pregnant.[2] It is estimated that 50 percent of teenagers who are 15 years of age are sexually active but only 10 percent utilize contraceptives within an average of one year after becoming sexually active.[3] Once teenage girls are faced with the reality of pregnancy, approximately 50 percent of these women give birth. Abortions account for 30 percent to 40 percent and the remainder result in miscarriage.[4]

The consequences of teenagers giving birth include educational, social, and economic disadvantages, resulting in increased health risks.[5,9] Risk factors include lack of knowledge and barriers to adequate health care services.[6] At the heart of the matter is the fact that many teenage mothers receive inadequate prenatal care, which leaves them and their babies at risk.[7] Approximately 50 percent of all pregnant teenagers receive no prenatal care during the first trimester.[8]

The South Florida Perinatal Network/Healthy Start Coalition for Dade County, established in 1979, focuses on the reduction of risk factors associated with ensured access to prenatal care for all pregnant women. In order to successfully implement such strategies, the contributions and insights of those people closest to the problem are needed. Thus, the coalition conducted a comprehensive Maternal and Infant Health Care Needs Assessment. Teenage Pregnancy was one area of focus and this paper highlights the needs assessment's relevant findings.[9]

Methods

Data were collected from the Florida Bureau of Vital Statistics. In addition, socioeconomic profiles at the zip-code level were extrapolated from commercially available census data for 76 zip codes in Dade County as well as 1990 census data. The Florida Bureau of Vital Statistics provided information regarding aggregate records of births registered in 1993; fetal death files; birth and death records of infants that died in 1993; and maternal characteristics used for the descriptive analysis provided in this report. Maternal characteristics such as mother's race (black, white, all others), ethnic origin (Hispanic, non-Hispanic), age group, and residential zip codes were provided in the descriptive analysis portion of the report. The data and profiles were validated using the following publications: *Florida Department of Health and Rehabilitative Services, Florida Vital Statistics Annual Reports* and *U.S. Department of Health and Human Services Annual Reports in Health United States*. More than 2,000 persons in Dade County contributed towards the development of the needs assessment report entitled The South Florida Perinatal Network/Healthy Start Coalition for Dade County, Maternal and Infant Health: Needs Assessment, December, 1994.

Findings

The total population of Dade county is 1,937,094, of which approximately 23 percent are women of childbearing age (aged 15-44).[9]

(continues)

Figure 11-1 The relationship between teenage pregnancy and poverty among Black teenagers.
Source: *Harvard Journal of Minority Public Health.*

Teenage Pregnancy and Poverty Among Black Teenagers

Table 1. Women of Childbearing Age (15–44) years

Age	1990 Census	1993 Estimate	2000 Projected
15–44	447,816	439,051	455,748
Total Female	1,008,625	1,017,282	1,103,761

Source: *Florida Population Studies, June 1994*

The racial configuration of Dade County is 73 percent white, 21 percent black, 0.2 percent Native American, 1.4 percent Asian/Pacific Islander, and 5 percent other.

Table 2. Race Distribution in Dade County and the State of Florida

	Total	White	Black	Native American	Asian/Pacific Islander	Other
Florida	12,937,926	10,749,285	1,759,534	36,335	154,302	238,470
Dade	1,937,094	1,413,015	397,993	3,066	26,307	96,713

Source: *1993 Florida Statistical Abstract*

In 1993, there were 2,592 teenage births in Dade County out of a total of 33,069 births.[9] Teenage pregnancies cross all racial and ethnic groups but the problem is disproportionately high among black teenagers in Dade County. Teenage births represent 7.8 percent of all Dade County live births with 12.7 percent among non-whites compared to 5.5 percent for whites.

Prenatal care was one of the primary issues considered in terms of teenage pregnancy. The Kessner Index is a composite index combining initiation of prenatal care, number of visits, and gestational term that was used to assess the adequacy of prenatal care.[10]

For all mothers, prenatal care was a greater problem among teenagers. Some (33 percent) received no care at all and others did not start care until the third trimester. In addition, teenagers were also at risk for insufficient levels of care. Of all teenage mothers, 23 percent had fewer than eight visits compared to 15.5 percent for mothers of all ages. Fifteen percent of teenage girls had six or fewer visits.

Another area of consideration was low birth weight, defined as affecting infants weighing 2500 grams or less. Young black mothers were at highest risk: 21.3 percent of their babies weighed less than 2500 grams at birth,

compared to a rate of 8.1 percent for the population at large.

Repeat pregnancies also present a particular problem for Dade County, Florida. The needs assessment indicates that of the 1,376 non-white girls who gave birth in 1993, 24 percent experienced a repeat pregnancy compared to 17 percent of the white teenage girls. Of those teens who delivered in 1993, 21 percent had other children at home. Data from the needs assessment indicate that at the time of delivery, 15 percent of all teenage girls in Dade County were married.

Discussion

Although no attempts were made to establish causalities in terms of the Maternal and Infant Needs Assessment of Dade County, certain factors relating to teenage pregnancy should be taken into consideration when reviewing the above findings.

First of all, there are apparent disparities in terms of black versus white teenagers in regard to teenage pregnancy. Black teenage girls are clearly overrepresented. Is it a matter of race, or should other factors be considered? In an effort to respond to this question it is necessary to take into consideration additional factors related to Dade County, Florida. The Dade County population totals approximately 1.94 million people. About 70 percent of

the population belongs to a racial or ethnic minority and the major ethnic influences are Cuba, Latin America, and the Caribbean.

Approximately 14.2 percent of Dade families live in poverty. Many of its low-income areas have high concentrations of minorities. The northern portion of the county, which includes the city of Opa-Locka and the areas of West Little River and Melrose are low-income designated concentration areas relevant to our discussion because they are also significant areas of racial and ethnic concentration in metropolitan Dade County. Large numbers of blacks also live in the Central Miami venues of Overtown, Liberty City, and other low-income areas.

This confluence of poverty and race is very telling. Black teenagers represent 14 percent of the United States teenage population. They are 2.5 times more likely to give birth and 5.5 times more likely to raise their children as single parents than are white teenagers.[1] Research indicates that some U.S. black teenagers living in poverty may view pregnancy as a symbol of achievement and as a boost to their self-worth. This perception may foster engagement in sexual intimacy.[11]

Poverty plays a recurring role in teenage parenting, particularly among black teenagers. Approximately 44.8 percent of black youths in the United States live below the poverty level and approximately 56 percent of blacks below the age of 25 live in inner cities.[13] Many black teenagers are living in substandard housing on streets that are crime-ridden, where they receive poor medical care and inadequate nutrition. Dade County is no exception.

A number of research studies regarding the issue of teenage pregnancy may shed some light on why black teenagers are overrepresented in terms of teenage pregnancy. It has been speculated that black teenagers living in poverty are more likely to have a fatalistic attitude as a result of a lifetime of economic deprivation and a sense of powerlessness to exercise control over their lives.[12] This attitude

Figure 11-1 *(Continued)*

may have some bearing on the fact that black teenage girls make the decision not to delay childbearing until their adult years.

In addition, pregnancy-prevention efforts in Dade County are fragmented and uncoordinated. There is no county-wide plan to address the problem. Teenage mothers in Dade County live primarily in areas where services are limited. Those individuals needing the services most do not have access to them. Another important factor is that most existing services are geared toward females. Outreach efforts are not sufficiently directed toward the young men who clearly are contributors to the problem of teenage pregnancy. Males need a range of similar preventive services to prevent unplanned pregnancy among teenagers.

Conclusions

It is clear that poverty is a major contributing factor to teenage pregnancy, particularly in regard to black girls. Thus, a need for more programs focusing on economic assistance, which foster independence is apparent. Programs should be readily accessible to at-risk teenage girls. It seems unlikely that programs will be successful if they are not accessible to those teenagers with the greatest need.

There is no doubt that poverty fosters feelings of powerlessness and hopelessness. For some poor teenagers, sexual relations, their pregnancies and having babies, may be seen as one of the few lifestyle options available which gives them direction and a sense of purpose. In addition, those teenagers who feel a sense of helplessness in their lives as a result of poverty and who have few educational goals tend to use contraception less effectively.[12, 14]

Thirty-one million Americans are without health care and adolescents are more likely to be uninsured than any other group. Inadequate health care means inadequate education in regard to contraception and information regarding pregnancy-resolution options.[15] Thus, an effort to reduce the occurrence of teenage pregnancy, particularly

amongst black teenagers must address many risk factors. Mechanisms need to be developed to help alleviate poverty and to enhance lifestyle options for black girls living in poverty. Black teenagers living in poverty must be provided with a way to see that the odds against them are manageable. Life skills must be taught to black teenagers in an effort to enhance their decision-making skills and to assist them in making logical and thoughtful decisions regarding pregnancy. Resources must be provided to help them to develop a level of competency regarding this issue and explore a myriad of positive options for their future and coping mechanisms must be put in place.

In addition, a nationwide effort must be made to provide comprehensive sex education, group and individual counseling, and medical contraceptive services. Dade County is taking significant steps to begin to deal with this problem beginning with the completion of the countywide needs assessment referred to above.

Success in reducing the incidence of teenage pregnancy, specifically in relationship to black teenagers in Dade County and nationwide, will necessitate the inclusion of community leaders, professionals, parents, religious and political leaders and what is most pivotal, the teenagers themselves—both males and females.

References

1. Frager, B. "Teenage Childbearing Part I: The Problem Has Not Gone Away." *Journal of Pediatric Nursing* 1991; 6: 131–133.

2. Leigh, BC, Morrison, DM, Trocki, K, et al. "Sexual Behavior of American Adolescents: Results from a National Survey." *Journal of Adolescent Health* 1994; 15: 117–125.

3. Gotlieb, E. *Practicing Adolescent Medicine: A Collection of Resources.* Elk Village, IL: American Academy of Pediatrics; 1994.

4. Stevens-Simons, C, and White, MM "Adolescent Pregnancy." Pediatric Annals 1991; 20:322–331.

5. Brown, S. "Can Low Birth Weight Be Prevented?" *Family Planning Perspectives* 1985; 17: 112–118.

6. Vincent, ML, Clearie, AF, and Schluchter, MD. "Reducing Adolescent Pregnancy Through School and Community Based Education." *Journal of the American Medical Association* 1987; 24: 3382–3386.

7. Makinson, C. "The Health Consequences of Teenage Fertility." *Family Planning Perspectives* 1985; 3:132–139.

8. Miller, DF *Dimensions of Community Health* Dubuque, IA: Brown and Benchmark. 1995.

9. South Florida Perinatal Network/ Healthy Start Coalition for Dade County. *Maternal and Infant Health: Service Gaps/Unmet Needs.* Dade County, FL: Florida's Healthy Start; 1994.

10. Kotelchuck, M. "An Evaluation of the Kessner Adequacy of Prenatal Care Index and a Proposed Adequacy of Prenatal Care Utilization Index." *American Journal of Public Health* 1994; 81:1414–1420.

11. Neal, EU, Jay and Litt, IF. "The Relationship of Self-Confidence and Autonomy to Oral Contraceptive Compliance Among Female Adolescents." *Journal of Adolescent Healthcare* 1985; 6:445–447.

12. Caldas, S. Current "Theoretical Perspectives On Adolescent Pregnancy and Childbearing On Adolescent Pregnancy and Childbearing in the United States." *Journal of Adolescent Research.* 1993; 8: 4–20.

13. Taylor, RL. Black "Youth: The Endangered Generation." *Youth and Society* 1990; 22: 4–11.

14. Holt, JL, and Johnson, SD. "Developmental Tasks: A Key to Reducing Teenage Pregnancy." *Journal of Pediatric Nursing* 1991; 3: 191–196.

15. Feroli, KL, Hobson, SK, Miola, ES, et. al. "School-based Clinics: The Baltimore Experience." *Journal of Pediatric Health Care* 1992; 6: 127–131.

16. Kaplan, DW, "School-based Health Centers: Primary Care in High School." *Pediatric Annals* 1995; 4: 192–200.

Figure 11-1 *(Continued)*

interventions from a culturally competent vantage point. Most literature (from the past, at the time that the aforementioned article was written in 1994, until today) suggests that the best approach to resolving the issue of teenage pregnancy is to provide teenagers with information, provide contraception, promote abstinence, and enhance decision-making skills. All of these suggestions have contributed to improvement since 1994, as overall in the United States, teenage pregnancy rates have declined. However, within the context of cultural competence, particularly when vast demographic changes are taking place, it is important for public health practitioners and other members of the healthcare field who work closely with teenage girls of color to approach this scenario from a culturally competent vantage point.

Although the article highlighted in this chapter focused on Black/African American girls in Dade County, Florida, at the time the article was written, approximately 70% of the population belonged to a racial or ethnic minority, with the major groups being Latin American (primarily but not exclusively Cuban), African American, and Caribbean. This demographic composition remains the same in Dade County today and is the direction, in terms of diversity, that communities throughout the United States are heading, particularly in urban areas. Therefore, an approach to dealing with teenage pregnancy, beyond what is delineated in the article, which identified poverty as the critical factor, is to use some of the cultural competence approaches discussed in previous chapters to communicate with young women of color about teenage pregnancy. These approaches could include the following:

- Ensuring that public health and healthcare organizations that intend to address the issue of pregnancy among teenage girls from minority groups understand the correlation between poverty and teenage pregnancy and that it is not relegated to a matter of race. For example, the statement that teenage pregnancy occurs among Black teenage girls more than any other groups may imply wanton promiscuity rather than an understanding of the confluence of poverty and sexual behavior among teenage girls in general.
- Using visual affirmation in developing informational materials for teenage girls from various racial groups. For example, pamphlets and other written materials, public service announcements, films, and other educational interventions should be designed including images that reflect the racial groups of the teenage girls. A teenage pregnancy prevention effort targeted to African American girls should present images of African American girls, for Asian girls, Asian images (with accuracy in terms of nationality), etc.

- Linguistic competency should be incorporated into the process to ensure that girls are provided with information both verbally (**interpretation**) and written (**translation**) that they can understand in their primary language. Because teenage pregnancy is an issue that involves minors, steps should be taken to ensure parental involvement is included also using linguistically competent approaches.
- Rearing of children in multicultural environments often includes an "it takes a village approach," as implied in the article; hence, success in reaching them may necessitate including community, religious, and political leaders; professionals; and parents, as the teenagers themselves.

An understanding of the need for and application of cultural competence when trying to resolve public health issues is a necessary next step. Although the specific example of teenage pregnancy is being explored in this chapter, the suggestions concerning cultural competence initiatives are applicable to most public health concerns as they pertain to multiracial and ethnic populations.

WOMEN OF COLOR AS A SPECIAL NEEDS POPULATION

In terms of health care, women are considered a special needs population, along with other groups such as children, the uninsured, the chronically ill, the elderly, ethnic and racial minorities, the homeless, and migrants. These categories are not mutually exclusive. As a combination of two of the groups, women and ethnic and racial minorities, women of color have particular issues and concerns when seeking health care, as illustrated by the teenage pregnancy example, including a lack of cultural understanding by their healthcare providers. Women are minorities and, consequently, are denied resources and privileges including, but not limited to, economic opportunity, communicative self-representation, and preferred lifestyles (Balcazar, Balcazar, Taylor-Ritzler, & Keys, 2010). As pointed out by Balcazar et al., the term minority, as it is used in regard to women, is unique:

> Although the term minority is often equated with numbers of racial or ethnic populations based on a census (e.g. 12/1% African American; 12.5% Latino [U.S. Census Bureau, 2002]) from a representative theory perspective, numerical underrepresentation is not an intrinsic property of being a minority (Mpofu & Conyers, 2004). For instance, females comprise the larger proportion of people in most societies, yet

are defined as minorities in many cases because of their economic and social oppression defined as the first key characteristics of minority status (Solomon, 1995; Wilson, 1996). (p. 160)

Additionally, when exploring concerns relevant to women, it is necessary to understand the terms sex and **gender**. According to Jacobsen (2008):

> Sex refers to the biological classification of people as male or female based on genetics (the presence of XX or XY sex chromosomes) and reproduction anatomy. Gender refers to social, cultural and psychological aspects of being male or female and is shaped by the social and cultural environment and experience as well as biology. There is tremendous variability in the way individual women and individual men express their gender and in the way cultures define gender roles. (p. 70)

There is a great degree of variation in gender roles, and as a result, women may have limited power over their own bodies and may be precluded from making decisions about when to have babies and how many they should have. They may also experience violence, both sexual and nonsexual, with the former possibly leading to sexually transmitted diseases (Jacobsen, 2008). This powerlessness that women experience, which is partially due to their smaller size, tendency to be physically weaker than men (Jacobsen), and minority status, impacts the standard of medical care they receive. As stated by Jacobsen:

> The standard for medical care for women has historically been less than that of men. Until recently, Western medicine treated women as "small men." It is now recognized that women's bodies differ from that of small males. For example, for a long time no one realized that the prevalence of heart disease is similar in both sexes and that heart disease is the most common cause of death in both men and women in the United States. Because men are more like to have "dramatic" heart attacks with crushing chest pain some women often have subtle symptoms like feeling more tired than normal, doctors do not as easily recognize heart attacks in women. As a result, heart disease in women has traditionally been under diagnosed. (p. 71)

Clearly, there are health disparities based on gender. Table 11-1 provides an indication of further gender differences.

Another core issue for women is the lack of cultural competence of their healthcare providers. Women of color also experience **simultaneous oppression**, which is the "experience of multiple types of oppression as a single experience, which individuals of African descent experience daily in

Table 11-1 Comparison of Burden of Disease in Women and Men

Women are more likely than men to:	Men are more likely than women to:
Have cancers of the reproductive system	Have lung, bladder, mouth, esophageal, and stomach cancer
Have complications from sexually transmitted infections like chlamydia and gonorrhea	Become infected with trypanosomiasis, schistosomiasis, leishmaniasis, lymphatic filariasis, and other tropical infections
Develop vision problems related to glaucoma, cataracts, and trachoma	Commit suicide and have drug use disorders
Have Alzheimer's disease and other dementias	Develop liver disorders such as cirrhosis, hepatitis B, and hepatitis C
Die from diabetes	Have lung diseases like tuberculosis and chronic obstructive pulmonary disease (COPD)
Develop musculoskeletal disorders like rheumatoid arthritis and osteoarthritis	
Develop autoimmune diseases like lupus	
Develop iron deficiency anemia	

Source: Data from World Health Organization. (2004). *World health report 2004*. Retrieved November 24, 2009, from http://www.who.int/whr/2004/en/.

Western society" (Balcazar et al., 2010, p. 161). How can women of color be understood culturally so that service can be provided optimally without women feeling a lack of trust regarding the provision of health care and public health? The issues of cultural competence related to women of color will be explored in four hypothetical case studies that are based on actual events.

CASE STUDY 1

An African American woman enters a healthcare facility where she is to receive a magnetic resonance image (MRI) of her spine. She has long hair in the style known as locks. She is greeted by the receptionists and asked to have a seat in the waiting area until the technician is ready to see her. A White, male technician arrives to escort the woman in for the procedure and briefly discuss the process of the MRI with her. During his overview, he indicates to her that she will have to remove any metal objects (such as pins in her hair and jewelry) and that she should remove her hair for the process. The woman is appalled by his latter statement and indicates to him that her hair is her own and cannot be removed. He responds by stating that he has served a number of Black women who have weaves and other "false" hair often held in by pins, so he was basically taking a precaution. The woman is highly insulted and asks to speak to the administrator on duty. A White woman,

> *in an elegantly tapered suit, arrives, hears the concern, and explains to the African American woman that the technician meant no harm but it is the policy of the facility to be thorough with all patients in terms of the provision of information and that he was correct in inquiring about her hair in the manner that he did to ensure safety during the MRI process. She offers no apology and curtly responds, "I hope this resolves your concerns as he was merely following our required protocol." The African American woman responds with a disappointed and curt thank you and leaves the building promptly vowing never to return. She seeks her MRI at another facility.*

In reviewing this case, one may not detect the gravity of the cultural insult that occurred and why the woman found it so offensive. However, for women of African descent, throughout the diaspora, hair is a critical aspect of their culture. The depth of the concern has historical implications. Through the atrocity of the slave trade, most Black people who arrived in America were transported, against their will, mainly from the west coast of Africa. The removal of identity was a central function of the enslavement process. The whole issue of language and naming is so central to identity that slaves were not allowed to speak their native language or maintain traditional names. The cultural genocide began as soon as captors collected slaves and could also be referred to as cultural destructiveness, per the Cultural Competence Continuum, as discussed in Chapter 5. On the ships during the unsavory voyage to the New World, slaves who spoke the same language or had the same markings of scarification were separated. Once in America, slave owners would not permit drumming because they knew slaves could communicate through the rhythms, another form of language.

Specific hairstyles of the slaves, in their home continent of Africa, were used to identify a geographic region. In the Wolof culture of Senegal, young girls partially shaved their hair as an outward symbol that they were not courting (Byrd & Tharps, 2002). The Karamo people of Nigeria were recognized for their unique coiffure—a shaved head with a single tuft of hair left on top (Byrd & Tharps). Widowed women would stop attending to their hair during their period of mourning so they would not look attractive to other men. Community leaders often donned elaborate hairstyles, and the royalty would often wear a hat or headpiece as a symbol of their stature. Africans from the Mende, Wolof, Yoruba, and Mandingo tribes often communicated age, marital status, ethnic identity, religion, wealth, and rank in the community through their ornate hairstyles.

The **Middle Passage** (which was the transport of slaves from Africa to the New World on slave ships across the Atlantic Ocean) and the slave trade destroyed this rich hair heritage of African people who were brought in as slaves to North America, the Caribbean, and Central and South America. Africans were no longer able to maintain elaborate hairstyles without their combs and herbal treatments used in Africa. Slaves relied on bacon grease, butter, and kerosene as hair conditioners and cleaners. From Ancient Egypt to West and East Africa, the hair of African people was (and still is) an adornment—both valued and appreciated. Unfortunately, Black hair was referred to as "wool" by the slave holders (Ivey, 2006); Whites looked upon Blacks who learned to style their hair like White women as "well adjusted." "Good" hair became a requirement to enter schools, churches, social groups, and businesses. In 1880, the hot comb was invented by the French. It was heated and used to straighten "kinky" hair. As time progressed, the hair of Black people was ridiculed and despised and referred to as buckwheat, kinky, nappy, bird feathers, and pickaninny (refers to a caricature of Black children of slaves and later African Americans that is widely considered racist) (Pilgrim, 2008). Rags or scarves were placed over the heads of Black women in books, films, and statuettes, and the women were referred to as mammies on television and in other forms of the media.

This painful history has caused many women of African descent to be extremely conscious and sensitive about their hair, and as a result, songs and poems have been written to help them to deal with this aspect of their lives. The famous singer India.Arie, after shaving her head completely in an effort to respond to the cultural indignation of her hair experiences throughout her career, said the following about her song "I Am Not My Hair":

> "As a Black American woman, a lot of your integrity is dictated by how you wear your hair," she explains. "The concept for the song was sparked when I decided to cut my locks, and all the different attitudes people had about it. This is my hair - and it's my life. I'll choose how I express myself." (India.Arie Biography, n.d.)

Many African American women have turned to weaves, extensions, and other remedies to address the hair issue. Others have turned to natural hairstyles. The natural hairstyles worn by African ancestors and some Black women today enabled/enable them to avoid scalp burns, hair breakage, and hair loss that often result from using harsh products to straighten their hair. As a result, some Black women of every generation have chosen to wear their hair naturally, regardless of trends, and natural hairstyles, such as locks, repeatedly resurface in the mainstream and are worn with extreme pride. Thus, healthcare providers should consider this history and the importance of hair for women of African descent as an example of an important cultural concept. Specifically, disregard for the importance of understanding the significance of an African American woman's hair and how to discuss it can lead to a serious cultural insult.

CASE STUDY 2

A Mexican woman is ready to deliver her baby in an American hospital. She is accompanied by her husband. The couple is monolingual Spanish speaking. She intends to have a vaginal delivery and is in extreme pain as a result of her contractions. Because her culture is very expressive, she loudly responds to pain during each contraction, and the nurses decide that perhaps her husband should come in the labor room to comfort her. They invite him in, and he comes in reluctantly and does not comfort his wife but sits very far away from her. The nurses, who are both non-Hispanic White women, are disgusted with him and go to find a Spanish-speaking nurse. The Spanish-speaking nurse is Cuban and approaches the man and begins to speak to him in harsh tones in Spanish asking why he will not attend to his wife. He does not respond and quietly sits there. The nurse walks away, and his wife continues to wail in pain without his assistance while the nurses try to comfort her. Eventually, the woman's mother arrives and comforts her daughter by wiping her brow, talking to her, and rubbing her back as the husband remains quietly seated across the room. The mother shows no animosity toward the husband for not assisting.

Culturally, there is a valid rationale for the behavior of the husband in this case. According to Galanti (2003):

> In Mexico, it is inappropriate for a husband to attend his wife during delivery. It is a woman's job, ideally the job of the mother. This may be due to the extreme modesty of Mexican women. American nurses who have difficulty believing that the modesty of Mexican women can extend to her own husband should be told of the eighty five year old Mexican woman with a tattoo of a small cross on her upper thigh. No one in her family—including her husband and daughters—had ever seen it. She told the nurse who was caring for her that she had done it in her wild and crazy youth. (p. 131)

Of course, it is important not to stereotype within a given culture because there may be variation within the Mexican culture regarding men attending to their wives during the birthing process, as well as variation among Black women regarding hair as discussed in the previous case. However, understanding cultural possibilities within various groups will help in ensuring that there is appreciation of scenarios that may not be understood by mainstream healthcare providers and public health practitioners. The lack of insight into the culture of the Mexican family in this case is clearly an indication of lack of cultural competence. One clear problem is assuming that a nurse who speaks Spanish will be able to comprehend the nature of the man's lack of involvement simply because they share a common language. Nationality matters regarding Hispanic people because cultures vary between Spanish-speaking countries. The nurse is Cuban, and the family is Mexican, and hence, they have two different cultures. Furthermore, the loud sounds made by the woman may not have been signs of distress, which was perhaps understood by her husband. Per Galanti (2003, p. 94), Mexican women often chant the phrase "aye yie yie" while in labor. What may appear to be an expression of pain might actually be a form of "folk Lamaze." Repeating the phrase in succession several times necessitates taking long, slow, deep breaths. Thus, it is a cultural method for alleviating pain.

Cultural understanding goes a long way in serving patients. Health service administrators and public health officials need to understand the importance of preparing staff and providers at every level in terms of dealing with cultural variations in a calm and comforting manner for both the patients/clients/customers and their families.

CASE STUDY 3

A child attending a school in a low-income community receives a pamphlet at her school that expresses the importance of reducing obesity and exercising. The child's school is having a problem in terms of increased levels of obesity and responds with a public health effort to try to communicate with the children and their parents. The goal is to initiate programs in the future in conjunction with a local public health entity in an effort to resolve the problem. The public health entity prepared an informative brochure for the school to distribute to the children so that the information could be shared with their parents. A child brings the pamphlet home to her mother and shares the information with her. After reviewing the brochure, the mother explains to her daughter that in her country where she was born and raised, South Africa, such matters of weight are not important. She advises her daughter that she is to eat heartily so that she is plump and healthy and that walking to and from school each day is sufficient exercise. She also points out to her daughter that the people depicted in the brochure are White, so the brochure is not for them but for other people. She throws the brochure in the garbage and tells her daughter to clean up and get ready for a hearty dinner, which she has prepared for the family so

> *that they can all be healthy and happy. Her husband works hard to ensure that they have plenty of food, which displays that they are doing well financially. She further advises her daughter to try and socialize with the other South African children at her school because there is a rather large, close-knit community of South Africans living in their community and attending her school and the South African children will better understand her.*

In this scenario, there is a disconnect between what is being shared with this particular parent through her child and the parent's cultural background. The perspective of the parent will impact how the child feels about the matter. As pointed out by Murthy and Smith (2009):

> In South Africa, it is a common belief among Black women that being overweight is a reflection of wealth and happiness. Many women residing in urban areas perceive body weight as an indication of their husband's ability to provide for their family. . . . Nearly half of all adult women in South Africa do not engage in enough exercise. Historically, women remained active while performing chores such as fetching water, tending to the animals and walking long distances. (p. 453)

Cultural beliefs are often maintained when South Africans, as well as other cultural groups that do not value being thin as a norm, travel to and live in the United States. Furthermore, the brochure developed by the public health organization does not visually affirm the woman and her daughter. The best approach by the public health entity and the school would be to conduct a demographic analysis of the students and parents to determine their race, ethnicity, and nationality. Once this is accomplished, information should be tailored for effective communication with the children and their parents. Perhaps the best approach for the South African family would be depictions of healthy, happy Black individuals presented in comfortable home environments. Reference could be made to the fact that quality of food, not quantity, can lead to a healthy lifestyle, including hearty portions of fruits, vegetables, and so on, to ensure that the suggestion is not to minimize the quantity of food eaten. The brochure could also include ideas of how to get exercise while conducting daily routines and perhaps present a table or figure paralleling routine activities (e.g., walking to school) with physical activities that may be conducted at the child's school in the gymnasium and on the playground. Basically, information must be presented in a manner that is congruent with the current understanding of the community and their unique cultural values.

Although it may not be possible or cost efficient to develop pamphlets tailored to meet the needs of every member of a given community, those groups with significant numbers must be addressed, or variations must be included to address the needs of diverse groups. For example, an array of images of various people from different races could be used, and information on various options in terms of foods to eat and types of exercise could be included. The outcome would be a culturally competent informational public health effort that speaks specifically to the needs of various segments of the community.

CASE STUDY 4

In a small community in New York City, on a street lined with Indian restaurants and saturated with the sounds and smells of India, a small group of women gather at a public health center where they have been invited to discuss contraception, spacing children, and limiting the number of births. The women are originally from a rural community in India called Utar Pradesh and have been in the United States for about a year. Their goal is to gain information so that they can share the process of contraception with their husbands. They understand that use of contraception would be breaking away from traditions in their home country and that their elders back in India and their husbands may not agree with it. However, after reviewing information that they acquired at a local community college, they are eager to learn more because they now live in the United States. Generally, the goal of young Indian women is to avoid multiple births that are spaced very closely. After several meetings and informative sessions at the public health center about contraception, the women share with the public health workers that although the information about contraception has been interesting, they will not be able to use contraceptives because their husbands do not agree and they will have too much difficulty explaining such a choice to their extended family. The public health workers realize that in every attempt that they have made to discuss and provide contraception to this particular cultural group, their success level is very low, and they are offered very little insight as to why from the participants.

Per Murthy and Smith (2009):

> Marriage in traditional India is not about individuals. It is a social contract between two families and an extremely important one because it brings two families together in a permanent bond. . . . Marriages are arranged between families that are similar to each other. Community caste and village of origin are the external flags that signal similarity

of overt parameters such as religion, language and food as well as inner parameters such as values and beliefs, customs and rituals, rules, norms and priorities. (p. 512)

Cultural competence becomes quite relevant in this scenario because it is important for public health practitioners who work with varying cultural groups to understand that success may not necessarily be gained by changing behaviors but merely in the provision of information so that individuals are in a position to make a decision. In this case, the cultural norm and long-term history of family in a community override an interest in change for the women. Information must also be presented to the public health workers regarding various aspects of Indian culture so that they can offer a culturally competent response to the women if their decision is contrary to the goal of the provision of contraception. As stated by Murthy & Smith (2009, p. 515) in a discussion of the dilemma that Indian women often face in regard to such matters, "It seemed easier by far to give in to the path of least resistance and have all the children that were wanted to complete the family." Furthermore, per National Family Health Survey, India (2004), in some instances in India, women will follow these births using terminal methods: "Female sterilization accounts for two-thirds of total contraceptive use and 77% of modern method use. Eighty-one percent of sterilized women were sterilized before age 30. The median age of sterilization is 25.5 years" (Murthy & Smith, 2009, p. 516). In general, there are a number of contraceptive options with varying pregnancy rates, as indicated in Table 11-2.

Again, this case exemplifies the need to understand unique characteristics of a given culture before trying to serve its members. Although success is not necessarily defined by the actions of the women in terms of contraception, the public health workers would have a better chance of communicating with them effectively and understanding their decision making if they had better insight into their culture.

CONCLUSIONS

Teenage pregnancy is a significant problem in the United States among women with a lower socioeconomic status. Although it superficially appears that race may be a factor in teenage pregnancy, the reality is that the overriding determinant is poverty, as indicated by the article entitled "The Relationship Between Teenage Pregnancy and Poverty Among Black Teenagers." Additionally, beyond teenage pregnancy, women of color are often misunderstood when seeking health care. The case studies in this chapter provide some insight regarding the importance of understanding

Table 11-2 Contraceptive Methods

Type	Approach	Approximate 1-year pregnancy rate	Sexually transmitted disease protection	Note
Complete abstinence	Abstinence	0%	Yes	No intercourse
Sterilization (tubal ligation or vasectomy)	Surgery	Nearly 0%	No	Permanent
Subdermal implants (Norplant)	Hormones	1%	No	Effective for about 5 years after implantation
Injection (Depo-Provera)	Hormones	1%	No	One injection every 3 months
Oral contraceptives	Hormones	1–2%	No	Pill must be taken daily to be effective
Transdermal (patch) contraceptives (Ortho Evra)	Hormones	1–2%	No	The patch must be replaced weekly
Intravaginal contraceptives (NuvaRing)	Hormones	1–2%	No	The vaginal ring must be replaced monthly
Emergency contraception ("morning after pill"/Plan B)	Hormones	—	No	Reduces pregnancy rate after unprotected sex from about 8% to about 2% if used within 72 hours of intercourse
Male condom	Barrier	11%	Yes	Apply just before intercourse
Diaphragm with spermicide	Barrier spermicide	6–20%	No	Inserted before intercourse
Sponge	Barrier	14–28%	No	Can be inserted before intercourse
Periodic abstinence	Timing	20%	No	Requires daily monitoring of body functions and periods of abstinence
Female condom	Barrier	21%	Some	Use just before intercourse
Spermicides	Spermicide	20–50%	No	Apply just before intercourse
No contraceptive method used	None	85%	No	

Sources: US Food and Drug Administration. (2003). *Birth control guide*. Retrieved November 24, 2009, from http://www.pueblo.gsa.gov/cic_text/health/birthcontrol/birthcontrolguide.html; Beers, M. H., & Berkow, R. (Eds.). (2006). Contraception. In, *The Merck manual of diagnosis and therapy* (18th ed.). Whitehouse Station, NJ: Merck Research Laboratory.

specific cultural nuances. By reviewing case studies, one can draw from the information and formulate ideas and insight in terms of handling similar matters pertaining to other groups and providing culturally competent health care to people from various racial, cultural, and ethnic groups while also considering their linguistic needs.

CHAPTER SUMMARY

Women are classified as a special needs population in health care. It should also be noted that women of color have additional needs that need to be considered in terms of their racial, ethnic, and cultural backgrounds to ensure that they are treated with dignity and not misunderstood. Issues such as teenage pregnancy among African American girls are explored in an effort to gain insight into how perceptions can be established as facts that are inaccurate and based on race without considering other determinants such as socioeconomic status.

Additionally, the case studies provide food for thought because some matters that may seem trivial to some people, such as African American hair, the intensity of a Mexican woman's expressions during labor and her husband's seeming lack of support, the perceptions of obesity of a South African woman, and a group of Indian women's decisions regarding contraceptives, may impact the perception of the efficacy of care and information provided of the people involved. However, in exploring these cases from a cultural competence vantage point, insight is gained, and a better understanding of the nuances of various cultures is the result.

CHAPTER PROBLEMS

1. Explain the relationship between teenage pregnancy, African American girls, and poverty, per the article discussed in this chapter.
2. Information is provided regarding the unique history of hair of African American women. Is this subject matter relevant to health care? If so, why should health service administrators and public health practitioners be aware of this history?
3. Unique insight was provided about certain aspects of what may happen in a labor and delivery scenario for a Mexican woman. Although none of the cultural information provided can be applied to Mexican women across the board, is such information useful for a healthcare organization that will be serving the Mexican population on a regular basis?

4. In reviewing all of the case studies, what is a common theme that one can garner from them? How are the case studies relevant to cultural competence?

5. Should women be considered as a special needs population in health care? Is it necessary to consider women of color further in terms of their race, culture, and ethnicity? Explain your responses thoroughly.

REFERENCES

Balcazar, F., Balcazar, Y., Taylor-Ritzler, T., & Keys, C. (2010). *Race, culture and disability: Rehabilitation science and practice.* Sudbury, MA: Jones and Bartlett Publishing.

Byrd, A., & Tharps, L. (2002). *Hair story: Untangling the roots of black hair in America.* New York: St. Martin's Griffin.

Galanti, G. (2003). *Caring for patients from different cultures.* Philadelphia: University of Pennsylvania Press.

India.Arie biography. Retrieved November 24, 2009, from http://www.contactmusic .com/info/india_arie.

Ivey, K. (2006). Combing the history of Black hair. *Sun-Sentinel,* February 21.

Jacobsen, K. (2008). *Introduction to global health.* Sudbury, MA: Jones and Bartlett Publishing.

Murthy, P., & Smith, C. (2009). *Women's global health and human rights.* Sudbury, MA: Jones and Bartlett Publishing.

National Family Health Survey, India. (2004). *Fertility and fertility preferences.* Retrieved September 5, 2009, from http://www.nfhsindia.org/data/ne/nechap4.pdf.

Pilgrim, D. *The picaninny caricature.* Ferris State University Museum of Racist Memorabilia. Retrieved March 2008, from http://www.ferris.edu/jimcrow/ picaninny.

Rose, P. (1998). The relationship between teenage pregnancy and poverty among Black teenagers. *The Harvard Journal of Minority Public Health.* III (I).

SUGGESTED READINGS

Francis, Z., & Francis, A. J. (2003). Fertility decline and gender bias in northern India. *Demography, 40*(4), 788–790.

Joubert, J., Norman, R., Lambert, E., Groenewald, P., Schneider, M., Bull, F., et al. (2007). Estimating the burden of disease attributable to physical inactivity in South Africa in 2000. *South African Medical Journal, 97,* 725–731.

United Nations. (2003). *Fertility, contraception and population policies.* Retrieved November 24, 2009, from http://www.un.org/esa/population/publications/ contraception2003/Web-final-text.PDF.

Viswanathn, H., Godfrey, S., & Yinger, N. (1998). *Reaching women: Unmet need for family planning in Uttar Pradesh, India.* Washington, DC: International Centre for Research on Women.

Cultural Competence Assessment Survey

EXECUTIVE TEAM AND MANAGEMENT

Site: _____

Date: _____

Please place a check mark ✓ next to the selection that best represents your thoughts.

1. I display pictures, posters, and other materials that reflect the cultures and ethnic backgrounds of patients/clients/customers who are served by my site.

   Strongly Agree ☐   **Agree** ☐   **Strongly Disagree** ☐   **Disagree** ☐   **N/A** ☐

2. I speak up when someone is humiliating another person or acting inappropriately.

   Strongly Agree ☐   **Agree** ☐   **Strongly Disagree** ☐   **Disagree** ☐   **N/A** ☐

3. I avoid using language that reinforces negative stereotypes.

   Strongly Agree ☐   **Agree** ☐   **Strongly Disagree** ☐   **Disagree** ☐   **N/A** ☐

4. I ensure that magazines, brochures, and other printed materials in reception areas reflect the different cultures of patients/clients/customers served by my site.

   Strongly Agree ☐   **Agree** ☐   **Strongly Disagree** ☐   **Disagree** ☐   **N/A** ☐

5. When using videos, films, or other media resources for health education, treatment, or other interventions, I ensure that they reflect the cultures of the patients/clients/customers served by my site.

   Strongly Agree □   **Agree** □   **Strongly Disagree** □   **Disagree** □   **N/A** □

6. I assist my new staff members, including people of various cultures, ages, and sizes, to feel welcome and accepted.

   Strongly Agree □   **Agree** □   **Strongly Disagree** □   **Disagree** □   **N/A** □

7. I disregard physical characteristics when interacting with others and when making decisions about competence and ability.

   Strongly Agree □   **Agree** □   **Strongly Disagree** □   **Disagree** □   **N/A** □

8. I am culturally competent.

   Strongly Agree □   **Agree** □   **Strongly Disagree** □   **Disagree** □   **N/A** □

9. I know the definition of cultural competence.

   Strongly Agree □   **Agree** □   **Strongly Disagree** □   **Disagree** □   **N/A** □

10. I know the definition of cultural proficiency.

    Strongly Agree □   **Agree** □   **Strongly Disagree** □   **Disagree** □   **N/A** □

11. I am culturally proficient.

    Strongly Agree □   **Agree** □   **Strongly Disagree** □   **Disagree** □   **N/A** □

12. I intervene in an appropriate manner when I observe my staff or patients/clients/customers engaging in behaviors that show cultural insensitivity or prejudice.

    Strongly Agree □   **Agree** □   **Strongly Disagree** □   **Disagree** □   **N/A** □

13. Cultural proficiency trainings/workshops will be helpful to my staff in their overall work performance.

    Strongly Agree □   **Agree** □   **Strongly Disagree** □   **Disagree** □   **N/A** □

14. My work responsibilities include direct patient/client/customer contact.

    Strongly Agree □   **Agree** □   **Strongly Disagree** □   **Disagree** □   **N/A** □

15. I have difficulty communicating with patients/clients/customers who cannot speak English.

    Strongly Agree ☐   **Agree** ☐   **Strongly Disagree** ☐   **Disagree** ☐   **N/A** ☐

16. All patients/clients/customers who visit my work site for service should know how to speak English if they want help.

    Strongly Agree ☐   **Agree** ☐   **Strongly Disagree** ☐   **Disagree** ☐   **N/A** ☐

17. Translation and signage should be available for patients/clients/customers with limited English proficiency (LEP).

    Strongly Agree ☐   **Agree** ☐   **Strongly Disagree** ☐   **Disagree** ☐   **N/A** ☐

18. Ongoing training and education for executives, management, and staff is necessary to promote cultural and linguistically competent/proficient service delivery.

    Strongly Agree ☐   **Agree** ☐   **Strongly Disagree** ☐   **Disagree** ☐   **N/A** ☐

19. I am interested in attending cultural competency/proficiency workshops/training sessions.

    Strongly Agree ☐   **Agree** ☐   **Strongly Disagree** ☐   **Disagree** ☐   **N/A** ☐

20. I use bilingual staff or trained volunteers to serve as interpreters during assessment, meetings, or events for patients/clients/customers who require this level of assistance.

    Strongly Agree ☐   **Agree** ☐   **Strongly Disagree** ☐   **Disagree** ☐   **N/A** ☐

Thank You

Cultural Competence Assessment Survey

STAFF

Site: _____

Date: _____

Please place a check mark ✓ next to the selection that best represents your thoughts.

1. I avoid imposing values that may conflict or be inconsistent with those of cultures of ethnic groups other than my own.
   Strongly Agree ☐   **Agree** ☐   **Strongly Disagree** ☐   **Disagree** ☐   **N/A** ☐

2. I speak up when someone is humiliating another person or acting inappropriately.
   Strongly Agree ☐   **Agree** ☐   **Strongly Disagree** ☐   **Disagree** ☐   **N/A** ☐

3. I avoid using language that reinforces negative stereotypes.
   Strongly Agree ☐   **Agree** ☐   **Strongly Disagree** ☐   **Disagree** ☐   **N/A** ☐

4. I get to know people from different groups and cultures as individuals.
   Strongly Agree ☐   **Agree** ☐   **Strongly Disagree** ☐   **Disagree** ☐   **N/A** ☐

5. I accept and reinforce the fact that not everyone has to act or look a certain way to be successful or valuable.
   Strongly Agree ☐   **Agree** ☐   **Strongly Disagree** ☐   **Disagree** ☐   **N/A** ☐

6. I assist new people at the site where I work, including people of various cultures, ages, and sizes, to feel welcome and accepted.

Strongly Agree ☐   Agree ☐   Strongly Disagree ☐   Disagree ☐   N/A ☐

7. I disregard physical characteristics when interacting with others and when making decisions about competence and ability.

Strongly Agree ☐   Agree ☐   Strongly Disagree ☐   Disagree ☐   N/A ☐

8. I am culturally competent.

Strongly Agree ☐   Agree ☐   Strongly Disagree ☐   Disagree ☐   N/A ☐

9. I know the definition of cultural competence.

Strongly Agree ☐   Agree ☐   Strongly Disagree ☐   Disagree ☐   N/A ☐

10. I know the definition of cultural proficiency.

Strongly Agree ☐   Agree ☐   Strongly Disagree ☐   Disagree ☐   N/A ☐

11. I am culturally proficient.

Strongly Agree ☐   Agree ☐   Strongly Disagree ☐   Disagree ☐   N/A ☐

12. I intervene in an appropriate manner when I observe other staff or patients/clients/customers within my work site engaging in behaviors that show cultural insensitivity or prejudice.

Strongly Agree ☐   Agree ☐   Strongly Disagree ☐   Disagree ☐   N/A ☐

13. Cultural proficiency trainings/workshops will be helpful to me in my overall work performance.

Strongly Agree ☐   Agree ☐   Strongly Disagree ☐   Disagree ☐   N/A ☐

14. My work responsibilities include direct patient/client/customer contact.

Strongly Agree ☐   Agree ☐   Strongly Disagree ☐   Disagree ☐   N/A ☐

15. I have difficulty communicating with patients/clients/customers who cannot speak English.

Strongly Agree ☐   Agree ☐   Strongly Disagree ☐   Disagree ☐   N/A ☐

16. All patients/clients/customers who visit my work site for service should know how to speak English if they want help.

Strongly Agree □   **Agree** □   **Strongly Disagree** □   **Disagree** □   **N/A** □

17. Translation and signage should be available for patients/clients/customers with limited English proficiency (LEP).

Strongly Agree □   **Agree** □   **Strongly Disagree** □   **Disagree** □   **N/A** □

18. Ongoing training and education for staff to promote culturally and linguistically competent/proficient service delivery is important.

Strongly Agree □   **Agree** □   **Strongly Disagree** □   **Disagree** □   **N/A** □

19. I am interested in attending cultural competency/proficiency workshops/training sessions.

Strongly Agree □   **Agree** □   **Strongly Disagree** □   **Disagree** □   **N/A** □

20. I recognize and challenge the biases that support my own thinking.

Strongly Agree □   **Agree** □   **Strongly Disagree** □   **Disagree** □   **N/A** □

Thank You

Cultural Competence Assessment Survey

PROVIDERS

Site: _____

Date: _____

Please place a check mark ✓ next to the selection that best represents your thoughts.

1. I display pictures, posters, and other materials that reflect the cultures and ethnic backgrounds of patients served by my site.

   Strongly Agree ☐ **Agree** ☐ **Strongly Disagree** ☐ **Disagree** ☐ **N/A** ☐

2. I make extra efforts to educate myself about the various cultures of my patients.

   Strongly Agree ☐ **Agree** ☐ **Strongly Disagree** ☐ **Disagree** ☐ **N/A** ☐

3. I avoid using language that reinforces negative stereotypes.

   Strongly Agree ☐ **Agree** ☐ **Strongly Disagree** ☐ **Disagree** ☐ **N/A** ☐

4. I ensure that magazines, brochures, and other printed materials in reception areas reflect the different cultures of patients served by my site.

   Strongly Agree ☐ **Agree** ☐ **Strongly Disagree** ☐ **Disagree** ☐ **N/A** ☐

5. When using videos, films, or other media resources for health education, treatment, or other interventions, I ensure that they reflect the cultures of the patient served by my site.

Strongly Agree □   **Agree** □   **Strongly Disagree** □   **Disagree** □   **N/A** □

6. I attempt to determine any family colloquialisms used by patients that may impact an assessment, treatment, or other intervention.

Strongly Agree □   **Agree** □   **Strongly Disagree** □   **Disagree** □   **N/A** □

7. I accept that religion and other beliefs may influence how families respond to illnesses, disease, and death.

Strongly Agree □   **Agree** □   **Strongly Disagree** □   **Disagree** □   **N/A** □

8. I am culturally competent.

Strongly Agree □   **Agree** □   **Strongly Disagree** □   **Disagree** □   **N/A** □

9. I know the definition of cultural competence.

Strongly Agree □   **Agree** □   **Strongly Disagree** □   **Disagree** □   **N/A** □

10. I know the definition of cultural proficiency.

Strongly Agree □   **Agree** □   **Strongly Disagree** □   **Disagree** □   **N/A** □

11. I am culturally proficient.

Strongly Agree □   **Agree** □   **Strongly Disagree** □   **Disagree** □   **N/A** □

12. I use bilingual staff or trained volunteers to serve as interpreters during assessment of patients who require this level of assistance.

Strongly Agree □   **Agree** □   **Strongly Disagree** □   **Disagree** □   **N/A** □

13. Cultural proficiency trainings/workshops will be helpful to me in the provision of health care.

Strongly Agree □   **Agree** □   **Strongly Disagree** □   **Disagree** □   **N/A** □

14. When possible, I ensure that all communiqués to patients are written in their language of origin.

Strongly Agree □   **Agree** □   **Strongly Disagree** □   **Disagree** □   **N/A** □

15. I have difficulty communicating with patients who cannot speak English

    Strongly Agree ☐ **Agree** ☐ **Strongly Disagree** ☐ **Disagree** ☐ **N/A** ☐

16. All patients who need care should know how to speak English if they want help.

    Strongly Agree ☐ **Agree** ☐ **Strongly Disagree** ☐ **Disagree** ☐ **N/A** ☐

17. Translation and signage should be available for patients with limited English proficiency (LEP).

    Strongly Agree ☐ **Agree** ☐ **Strongly Disagree** ☐ **Disagree** ☐ **N/A** ☐

18. Ongoing training and education for health providers is necessary to promote cultural and linguistically competent/proficient service delivery.

    Strongly Agree ☐ **Agree** ☐ **Strongly Disagree** ☐ **Disagree** ☐ **N/A** ☐

19. I am interested in attending cultural competency/proficiency workshops/training sessions.

    Strongly Agree ☐ **Agree** ☐ **Strongly Disagree** ☐ **Disagree** ☐ **N/A** ☐

20. I recognize that the meaning or value of medical treatment and health education may vary greatly among cultures.

    Strongly Agree ☐ **Agree** ☐ **Strongly Disagree** ☐ **Disagree** ☐ **N/A** ☐

Thank You

Glossary of Important Terms

A

Agency for Healthcare Research and Quality (AHRQ): One of 12 agencies within the Department of Health and Human Services. Its mission is to improve the quality, safety, efficiency, and effectiveness of health care for all Americans.

Alternative form reliability: The utilization of differently worded items to measure the same attribute.

American Medical Association (AMA): Organization that provides insight and information regarding the medical field and support for physicians. AMA also has a public health focus that entails promoting healthy lifestyles, providing resources for health professionals, and serving as a center for public health preparedness, disaster response, and vaccination resources. In general, it works to advance quality improvement in patient care.

Attitude-based approaches: Cultural competence training approaches that improve awareness of specific elements of attitudes, values, and beliefs regarding various cultures and of perspectives about language and other culturally and linguistically relevant factors that may impact the provision of optimal services to patients/clients/customers.

B

Bottom line: Net income of an organization.

C

Commission on Accreditation of Healthcare Management Education (CAHME): An accrediting body that sets criteria regarding healthcare management.

Construct validity: Asks the following question about an instrument: Does the instrument measure the theoretical framework that it is designed to measure?

Content validity: The sampling adequacy of the items used to measure the subject matter.

Convergent validity: Implies that several different methods for obtaining the same information about a given concept produce similar results.

Council on Education for Public Health (CEPH): Provides accreditation for institutions that prepare graduates for public health practice.

Criterion validity: Provides quantitative evidence of the accuracy of a survey instrument.

Cultural awareness: The ability of healthcare providers to appreciate and understand their clients' values, beliefs, life ways, practices, and problem-solving strategies.

Cultural blindness: Scenarios in which all people are viewed the same without taking into consideration that cultural differences matter.

Cultural competence: Cultural and linguistic competence is a set of congruent behaviors, attitudes, and policies that come together in a system, agency, or among professionals that enables effective work in cross-cultural situations. Per the Cultural Competence Continuum, cultural competence involves ensuring that the needs of diverse patients/clients/customers are met by health service and public health organizations based on the acquisition of specific skill sets, valuing diversity, and taking concrete steps to ensure efficacy in serving minority populations.

Cultural desire: The ability of the healthcare provider/health service administrator/public health practitioner to possess a drive to achieve cultural competence.

Cultural destructiveness: Attitudes, policies, practices, and structures within a system or organization that are destructive to a cultural group.

Cultural encounters: The ability of healthcare providers to competently work directly with clients of culturally diverse backgrounds. This is demonstrated by verbal and nonverbal messages by the healthcare provider and the patient/client/customer.

Cultural filtration: When cultural beliefs or ideas are either included or removed from the interpretation process by the interpreter.

Cultural incapacity: The lack of capacity to respond effectively to culturally and linguistically diverse groups.

Cultural knowledge: Insight and knowledge about physical, physiologic, and biologic variations among groups and about various cultures.

Cultural nuances: Subtle differences between particular cultures.

Cultural precompetence: When a healthcare organization is aware of its strengths and areas for growth and there is a clear commitment to human and civil rights.

Cultural proficiency: Takes the process of cultural competence a step further by employing staff and consultants with cultural expertise, ensuring assessment and training efforts, and reviewing policies and procedures to ensure the inclusion of culturally competent language.

Cultural sensitivity: An awareness of and respect for a patient's cultural beliefs and values.

Cultural skill: The ability of healthcare providers to conduct an accurate and culturally competent history and physical examination.

Culturally and Linguistically Appropriate Services (CLAS) standards: The purpose of the CLAS standards is to address the inequities that exist in the provision of health care and to make services more responsive to the individual needs, on a cultural and linguistic basis, of patients/clients/consumers served.

Culture: An integrated pattern of learned beliefs and behaviors that can be shared among groups including thoughts, styles of communicating, ways of interacting, views on roles and relationships, values, practices, and customs.

D

Divergent validity: Assessed by comparing a respondent's answer to a question measuring one concept to their answer to a question intended to measure a different concept; if divergent validity is present, the answers will be different.

Diversity: The makeup of the workforce of a given healthcare organization; this includes ethnic and racial backgrounds, age, physical and cognitive abilities, family status, sexual orientation, socioeconomic status, religious and spiritual values, and geographic location and all of the dimensions and differences between people.

E

Emerging majorities: A terms used to describe an inevitable change taking place in American society based on the prediction that by the year 2050, in certain geographic areas in the United States, the majority populations will be Hispanics and Blacks and other minorities (combined) and Whites will be the minority group.

Ethnicity: A group or individual's conception of cultural identity, which includes a wide variety of learned behaviors that a human being uses in his or her natural and social environment to survive that may result in cultural demarcation between and within societies.

F

Face validity: Entails a review of the items of a survey by individuals who are not trained in the survey development process.

G

Gender: "Gender refers to social, cultural and psychological aspects of being male or female and is shaped by the social and cultural environment and experience as well as biology. There is tremendous variability in the way individual women and individual men express their gender and in the way cultures define gender roles." (Jacobsen, 2008, p. 70)

H

Health disparity: Healthcare inequality or gaps in the quality of health and health care across racial, ethnic, and socioeconomic groups and population-specific differences in the presence of disease, health outcomes, or access to health care.

I

Informed consent: Consent by a patient to a surgical or medical procedure or participation in a clinical study after achieving an understanding of the relevant medical facts and the risks involved.

Institute of Medicine (IOM): The IOM is a component of the National Academy of Sciences, and its purpose is to advise the nation about health, biomedical science, and medicine.

Internal consistency: A measure of reliability that is a determination of the performance levels of various aspects of the same concept.

Interpretation: To turn oral/spoken words into one's own or another language.

J

The Joint Commission: The accrediting body for healthcare organizations, including hospitals, community health centers, and other types of healthcare facilities.

K

Knowledge-based approaches: Cultural competence training approaches that include specific information of relevance to cultural competence, including definitions of culture, race, ethnicity, linguistic competence, and related concepts; details about health-seeking behaviors of various cultures; and so on.

L

Lack of clarity: Refers to whether or not the questions in a survey are vague or ambiguous.

Lack of complexity: How easy an instrument is to administer.

Linguistic competence: The capacity of an organization and its personnel to communicate effectively and convey information in a manner that is easily understood by diverse audiences including persons of limited English proficiency, those who have low literacy skills or are not literate, and individuals with disabilities, and the ability to communicate effectively and accurately with individuals whose primary language is not English.

M

Mainstream: A term that is often used to describe the "general market" and usually refers to a broad population that is primarily White and middle class.

Malpractice: Improper or negligent treatment of a patient, as by a physician, resulting in injury, damage, or loss.

Middle Passage: The transport of slaves from Africa to the New World on slave ships across the Atlantic Ocean.

Mission (of an organization): A brief statement that indicates why the organization exists and states the purpose of the organization.

N

Nationality: An identity that can be defined by a person's place of legal birth or by a person's associational citizenship status governed by where an individual resides and works, which may defy national boundaries and sovereignty.

P

Paradigm shift: A revolutionary change from one way of thinking to another, which does not just happen but is driven by agents of change.

People of color: Individuals who are classified as being part of minority groups, namely, Blacks or African Americans, Native Americans, Alaska Natives, Asians and Pacific Islanders, and Hispanics or Latinos.

R

Race: Biologic variation including phenotypical differences in stature, skin color, hair color, facial shape, and other inherited characteristics that may or may not be mutually exclusive in each individual.

Reliability (of a survey): The stability and equivalence of measures of the same concept over time or across methods of gathering data.

Return on investment: The monetary benefits derived from having spent money on developing or revising a system.

S

Simultaneous oppression: The "experience of multiple types of oppression as a single experience, which individuals of African descent experience daily in Western society." (Balcazar et al., 2010, p. 161)

Skill-building approaches: Cultural competence training approaches that develop specific skill sets that will prepare individuals with knowledge of how to communicate effectively with individuals who do not speak English, how to identify an interpreter when needed, and how to ensure that individuals feel valued and appreciated in terms of their culture based on discussions with them about cultural nuances when they enter a healthcare or public health facility.

Stereotypes: Exaggerated beliefs or fixed ideas about a person or group of people.

Sullivan Commission: The Sullivan Commission is primarily a diversity initiative and attempts to reduce racial and ethnic disparities through increasing diversity in the health professions.

T

Test–retest reliability: Conducted to determine whether an instrument will measure what it is purported to measure, from time 1 to time 2.

Translation: To turn the written word into one's own or another language.

V

Validity: The consistency of the results of a measure.

Visual affirmation: The physical surroundings of healthcare organizations, such as artwork and images, that reflect the patients/clients/customers served.

W

Wisdom of crowds: Collective predictions or a collaborative filter.

Web Sites and Resources

CULTURAL COMPETENCE AND OTHER RELEVANT WEB SITES

American College of Healthcare Executives: http://www.ache.org

American Medical Association, Culturally Effective Health Care: http://www.ama-assn.org/ama/pub/about-ama/our-people/member-groups-sections/minority-affairs-consortium/news-resources/culturally-effective-health-care.shtml

American Medical Student Association, Health Equity Scholars Program: http://www.amsa.org/AMSA/Homepage/EducationCareerDevelopment/AMSAAcademy/HealthEquityScholarsProgram.aspx

American Public Health Association: http://www.apha.org

Commission on the Accreditation of Healthcare Management Education (CAHME): http://www.cahme.org

Council of Education for Public Health: http://www.CEPH.org

CulturedMed: https://culturedmed.sunyit.edu/index.php/cultural-profiles

DiversityRx, L-E-A-R-N Model of Cross Cultural Encounter Guidelines for Health Practitioners: http://www.diversityrx.org/HTML/MOCPT2.htm

Institute of Medicine: http://www.IOM.edu

Office of Minority Health: http://www.omhrc.gov/

Office of Minority Health, National Standards on Culturally and Linguistically Appropriate Services (CLAS): http://www.omhrc.gov/templates/browse.aspx?lvl=2&lvlID=15

Office of Women's Health Cultural Competence: http://www .womenshealth.gov/health-professionals/cultural-competence/index.cfm

The Joint Commission: http://www.jointcommission.org

US Department of Health and Human Services: www.hhs.gov

JOURNAL ARTICLES AND BOOKS

See also the Suggested Readings at the end of each chapter.

American Academy of Pediatrics Committee on Community Health Services. (1997). Health care for children of immigrant families. *Pediatrics, 100*(1), 153–156.

Betancourt, J. (2003). Cross cultural medical education: Conceptual approaches and frameworks for evaluation. *Academic Medicine, 78*(6), 560–569.

Boedigheimer, S., & Gebbie, K. (2001). Currently employed public health administrators: Are they prepared? *Journal of Public Health Management and Practice, 7*(1), 30–36.

Boult, L. (1995). Underuse of physician services by older Asian-Americans. *Journal of the American Geriatrics Society, 43*(4), 408–411.

Brach, C., & Fraser, I. (2002). Reducing disparities through culturally competent health care: An analysis of a business case. *Quality Management in Health Care, 10*(4), 15–28.

Byrd, W., & Clayton, L. A. (1992). An American health dilemma: A history of blacks in the health system. *Journal of the National Medical Association, 84,* 189–200.

Collins, K., Hughes, D., Doty, M., Ives, B., & Edwards, J. (2002). *Diverse communities, common concerns: Assessing health care for minority Americans. Findings from Commonwealth Fund 2001 Health Care Quality Survey.* New York: Common Wealth Fund Publication.

Cooper, L. (2003). Patient-centered communication, ratings of care and concordance of patient and physician race. *Annals of Internal Medicine, 139,* 907–916.

Davidhizar, R., Dowd, S. B., & Giger J. N. (1998). Educating the culturally diverse healthcare student. *Nurse Education in Practice, 23*(2), 38–42.

DeGenova, M. (1997). *Families in cultural context: Strengths and challenges in diversity.* Mountain View, CA: Mayfield Publishing Co.

DeLew, N., & Weinick, R. (2000). An overview: Eliminating racial, ethnic and SES disparities in health care. *Health Care Financing Review, 21*(4), 1–7.

Dengler, C. (1995). *Cultural competence: Program self-assessment. Services to children and families.* St. Paul, MN: Amherst H. Wilder Foundation.

Deters, K. (1997). Belonging nowhere and everywhere: Multiracial identity development. *Bulletin of the Menninger Clinic, 61*(3), 368–384.

Helman, C. (1990). *Culture health and illness* (2nd ed.). Oxford, England: Butterworth-Heinemann.

Hufford, D. (1997). Folk medicine and health culture in contemporary society. *Primary Care, 24*(4), 723–741.

Institute of Medicine. (2003). *Who will keep the public healthy? Educating public health professionals for the 21st century.* Washington DC: The National Academies Press.

Levine, M. (1997). Exploring cultural diversity. *Journal of Cultural Diversity, 4*(2), 53–56.

Mason, J. (1995). *The Cultural Competence Self-Assessment Questionnaire: A manual for users.* Portland, OR: Portland Research and Training Center.

Mateo, M., & Smith, S. (2001). Workforce diversity: Challenges and strategies. *Journal of Multicultural Nursing and Health, 7*(2), 8–12.

Randall-David, E. (1989). *Strategies for working with culturally diverse communities and clients.* Bethesda, MD: The Association for the Care of Children's Health.

Shah, S. (1998). The ethnic minority traveler. *Infectious Disease Clinics of North America, 12*(2), 523–541.

Spector, R. (1991). *Cultural diversity in health and illness* (3rd ed.). Norwalk, CT: Appleton and Lange.

Thiederman, S. (1996). Improving communication in a diverse healthcare environment. *Healthcare Financial Management, 50*(11), 72, 74–75.

Tirado, M. (1996). *Tools for monitoring cultural competence in health care.* San Francisco: Latino Coalition for a Healthy California.

Ward, R. (1998). Understanding and embracing multiculturalism in the health care arena. *Michigan Medicine, 97*(5), 24–31.

Weaver, H. (1998). Indigenous people in a multicultural society: Unique issues for human services. *Social Work, 43*(3), 203–211.

Whyte, S. R. (1998). Help for people with disabilities: Do cultural differences matter? *World Health Forum, 19*(1), 42–46.

Yee, D., & Tursi, C. (2002). Recognizing diversity and moving toward cultural competence: One organization's effort. *Generations, 26*(3), 54–58.

Youdelman, M., & Perkins, J. (2002). *Providing language interpretation services in health care settings: Examples from the field. The Commonwealth Fund, Field Report.* Retrieved November 29, 2009, from http://www.commonwealthfund.org/usr_doc/youdelman_languageinterp_541.pdf?section=4039.

Cultural Competence Plan

Company Analysis

Brief Organizational History with Cultural Competence Emphasis

Community Analysis

Local demographics

Patient/client/customer demographics

Staff demographics

Executive and management demographics

Board of directors demographics

Provider demographics

Cultural Competence Assessment

Board and executive team

Providers

Staff

Facility Assessment (Visual Affirmation and Bilingual/ Multilingual Signage)

Waiting areas

High-traffic areas

Staff-accessible areas

Reading materials and written information

Web site review

Review of procedures, protocols, and mission and vision statements

Strategic Cultural Competence Marketing Plan and Development

Strategic Approach

Expected cultural competence goals and outcomes

Achieving diversity

Cultural competence champions (committee)

Internet cultural marketing and training

Community Partnering

Community leaders

Key organizations

Supporting affiliates/stakeholders

Cultural Competence Project Timeline

Key elements

Key points and dates

Check points

Postproject Assessment/Evaluation

Goal measurement

Continued cultural competence assessment (ongoing)

Index